L.A. Book Fair 2017

Diane —

The pedigree of a . . .

PARAMEDIC HERETIC

Immutable Laws and Ethical Illusions

Terrific to meet you — Stay safe —

K. Patrick McDonald

By K. Patrick McDonald

First published by Dog Ear Publishing
4010 W. 86th Street, Ste H
Indianapolis, IN 46268
www.dogearpublishing.net

ISBN: 978-1-4575-3180-4

Library of Congress Control Number: has been applied for

This book is printed on acid-free paper.

Printed in the United States of America

"We are indebted to Mr. McDonald's research, as well as numerous extraordinary cases brought to our attention over the years."

—David Muir and Elizabeth Vargas, Investigative Reporters
ABC's *20/20 News Magazine*

❖

"From ego-errors and tomfoolery, to greed, stupidity and murder – I've laughed and cried at McDonald's astutely biting, at times hysterical view of my peer-group. His observations are disturbing, provocative and when you least expect it, uncomfortably funny."

—Lesley Miller, MD retired (former *"Surgeon to the Stars"*)
USC School of Medicine, Los Angeles

❖

"We're not here to denigrate health care workers. They have dedicated their lives to treating human suffering and they're overworked. But I happen to be a pilot as well as an actor, and I can promise you there is a reason that flying a commercial airliner today is safer than hospitals. It's because when an air accident happens, the NTSB jumps on it instantly and does not quit until they figure out what happened. They hide nothing. Warts and all, they make their findings public. That is exactly what Mr. McDonald does; exactly what health care in America desperately needs. These things have got to change."

—Dennis Quaid, Actor, Health Care Activist
Created the *Quaid Foundation*, after his twins babies
nearly died from an accidental overdose in a hospital

"En Vino, Veritas"

In wine there is truth

Pliny the Elder, Roman Historian

❖

"To reach the wine in health care, you must outsmart the serpent"

The Author

Contents

This book is dedicated to . . .

Jerry & Yvonne DeBolt
Gary Smith & Jerriann Dalman
Louann DeBolt & Eddie Lowery
Ed & Diane Pendleton
&
Roxanne

. . . the most decent and generous people I know

Forewords

As a young practitioner I was among a small group of doctors in the 1950s to recognize that caring for the sickest patients required a change in the way care was delivered. More than anything else, this meant a change in our thinking. Not all of my colleagues agreed.

The author here, I suspect, is not far astray when he submits there need to be changes in the way pre-hospital care is delivered, too. And it is fair to surmise that not all of his colleagues will agree, either. In my view, Mr. McDonald's 30-year EMS career success – much of it right here in the Coachella Valley, by the way – lays ample foundation for him to turn his stethoscope onto those aspects of health care in serious need of attention. His research alone causes me to share his dismay, particularly with his findings of widespread physician misbehavior. It is a sad state of affairs that Paramedics might – even for an instant – distrust the very caregivers they turn their patients over to. I am a doctor, after all, and I don't like this one bit. I confess this matter eluded me for an entire career and I regret it.

With health care front and center in today's headlines, Mr. McDonald's voice is an important one, now more than ever. He reveals a number of disturbing realities. We might want to pay close attention to what this gentleman has to say.

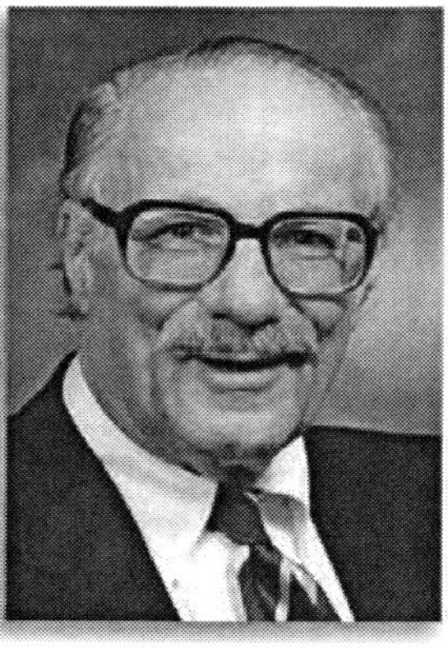

Doctor Max Harry Weil
Founder, *Weil Institute of Critical Care Medicine*
Considered the "Father" of Critical Care Medicine

I recall first meeting the author, back in the early years of the San Diego EMS system. "Paramedics" were a new species then and I'd never met one. I was sitting at my desk at the television station one morning when he walked into my office and asked me point blank how much I knew about the "strain of insanity" in rescue politics. He wore an impeccable white uniform shirt with a gold nametag; a patch on each shoulder and an intense expression. I told him I had very little time to discuss much of anything at the moment, but if he made an appointment we could probably chat someday. He sat down across from me anyway, leaned forward in his seat, and proceeded to school me on a fascinating subject about which I knew absolutely nothing. The extent of my ignorance – and the depth of his passion – captivated me enough that an hour later he was still talking and I sat scribbling notes like a kid in a classroom. I was so intrigued that I invited him to do a series of commentaries at the end of our newscasts and he agreed. We never regretted it. Patrick McDonald knew what he was talking about then and he is wiser now. He writes books these days and for my money, we are immensely better for it.

As a career newsman I've always had a keen interest in pertinent social issues. And I cannot think of a more pressing issue of our time than the dangers lurking in U.S. health care. After all, at some point we are all patients, and Patrick does an admirable job of arming us with an oft-forgotten weapon: logic.

So read what he says. *Consider how it impacts your family.* His observations will make you smarter, as they have surely made me. And don't be surprised if what you learn from him saves your life someday.

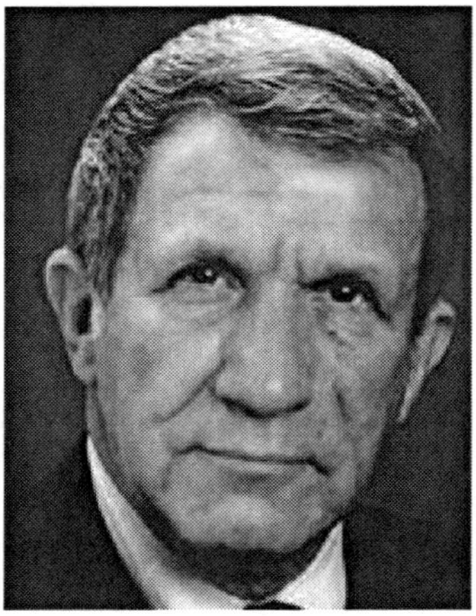

Carl Sisskind
Editorial Director,
KFMB-TV News 8
San Diego *CBS* affiliate
(Retired)

Prologue

Here's an idea. Let's have a little chat. Pretend you and I are stuck in an elevator for a few hours. No one else around. So we slump to the carpeted floor, lean back against the walls and try to get comfortable. We take judicious sips of our handy bottles of water and start comparing life notes, just you and I. We flip a coin; you win the toss, so I have to go for first . . . .

❖

It would have been more fun to pen one of those feel-good books so readily found on the non-fiction shelves at *Barnes & Noble*. After all, they certainly do seem to sell. You know the ones. Books that trumpet rescue heroics: our exciting, daily battles against the devil's own work of trauma and disease. Those breathless first-person accounts regaling readers of our wondrous deeds, like breathing air into a lifeless baby by the pool; reviving a grandfather against frangible odds; snatching tenuous lives from the jaws of an ugly death. The Grim Reaper shows up with his nasty scythe to do the deed. Paramedics fight him off with needles and drugs and unparalleled street-smarts.

A common theme found in these tales – and you see it both in print and on film – is that of the steely-eyed lifesaver, bravely ignoring vapid protocols and overbearing, perhaps even witless superiors, to strike out on a shaky limb and just do the right thing. After all, what rescuer worth his sodium isn't willing to roll the dice? We're *saving lives* here. What could be more important? Of course, at the satisfying conclusion of these stories to almost no one's surprise, a few sad souls have died, but most patients survive to smile through grateful tears. And then on cue our hero stands bloody but forgiven, his or her left-field antics and heat-of-the-crisis vitriol forgotten or – even more vacuous – admired. Because in the end, with all the false modesty our rescuer can muster, we as a dependent society need – no, strike that, *demand* – to be spoon-fed these inevitable words:

"We aren't really heroes. We just did what we're trained to do."

Indeed, of all our earthly endeavors, surely rescue is the singular place – is it not? – where heroic ends justify any means. A realm where key players on the lifesaving stage put aside their *Grey's Anatomy, Chicago Fire* and *Trauma: Life in the ER* differences when it matters; actually pool their brilliance long enough to place the glorious effort of retrieving human lives above all else.

And you believe this, right?

Well, you might want to hold your ponies.

You see, our dispute with these 'feel-good' narratives is in their deception of the citizenry. You and your families rely on truth in advertizing and you are assuredly not getting it. These stories reinforce your already flawed assumption that when it comes to medicine, Americans have at least one safe haven to count on. So the end result is a Band Aid on cancer. In our era of so many important social machinations already in disarray, the authors of these books conveniently, deftly sidestep the fact that health care gone wrong is the single most lethal creature in our societal sea of serpents. Why do we pretend it isn't so? Because it is quite literally miserable to even think about. When it comes to health care, we as providers cling to the same warm trumpery that you do – namely, that what we do is overwhelmingly ethical and good. Epiphanies can hit you like a pie in the face, so we avoid them whenever we can. As a tiny example, consider this little oddity:

The original insignia of medicine – the *Rod of Asclepius* – has long since been replaced in the U.S. by the symbol of trickery and commerce, thieves and liars – the *caduceus*. What a pluperfect harbinger of the status quo that turned out to be. Listen, if you will, to these words:

"How can we trust a profession that cannot even get its symbols straight? Most physicians in the United States think the symbol of their profession is something called the caduceus. Not true. Historians have discovered that someone in the Army Medical Corps mistook the caduceus for the Rod of Asclepius more than 100 years ago. Not long after, every doctor in America was emulating the mistake."

—Daniel Sulmasy MD
University of Chicago Medicine Ethics

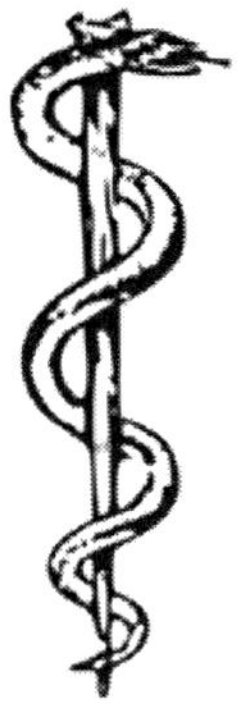

Rod of Asclepius

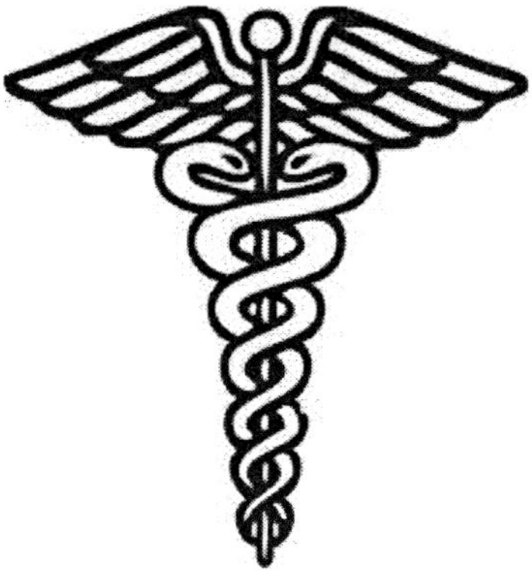

Caduceus

But when we double the serpents, don't we double the venom?

Within London's Guildhall Museum I once stood and stared at a tiny container seal on display, circa 3rd Century, caduceus emblem clearly defined. Historians at the Guildhall believe the symbol was in that era used in reference to the writings of Homer, the Greek author and poet. Homer was a pretty bright fellow. He recognized the doubled serpent caduceus was the enterprise of sorcerers and witches, "possessing the ability to charm the eyes of men."

It certainly charmed me. While still in school I spent money that should have been saved. I went out and bought an exquisite,18-karat gold caduceus for my collar, thereby adopting the very absurdity of the physician professors around us. With so much to master in too short a time in this business, the reflex is to unthinkingly ape the behavior around you. So we do exactly that.

Now the truth is, for any medic with a three-decade, 20,000+ emergency response history, populating yet another book with poignant rescue sagas would be surprisingly easy. We all have war stories to tell – from the hilarious to the homicidal – and some of them are truly riveting. Those of us who have labored in the 911 trenches have indeed saved lives while risking our own, and even though we don't say it in front of the cameras, plenty of us believe we are heroes. Just ask the patients. That wasn't Spiderman swinging off the rooftop to pull them from the burning motor home. It wasn't Robocop catching their drugged-up teenager by the pants leg, as he dove out the hotel window. So of course we save lives and we are damned proud of it. The point here is not to say the feel-good books are inherently wrong.

What they are is invariably myopic. They paint the picture that – with rare exception – health care is overwhelmingly guileless. And that is regrettably, verifiably not true. The patient care industry has long since been compromised by an utter disregard for its own chicanery. The medical arts have successfully managed to shroud their sins and shuffle their sinners. Too much of the probity of health care is woefully undeserved.

Put it this way: as long as American medicine is allowed to hide its demons, it is naïve – more, it is stupid – for a populace to view its practitioners and managers as invariably altruistic. Make no mistake. The gallimaufry of medicine has always engendered a fertile ground for capitalistic predators. It provides terrific niches for off-the-chart sociopaths. And too many of us who are not, have become ingeniously adept at hiding those who are. Paramedics are particularly guilty of willful ignorance. I should know. For decades, my silence cloaked as many scoundrels as anybody's.

At some point in life – should you harbor an inkling of ethics – you step outside yourself. You appraise your body of work and make the painful decision to balance the slate. You do all in your power to drive a wooden stake through the heart of the camorra. You tell the truth.

I wasn't always a heretic, of course. In my salad days I was as blissfully ignorant as interns tend to be, cheerfully willing to chomp onto the shiny, enticing fishhook called 'rescue' with no fear of consequence. Newbie's to most professions are sodden with more limerence than common sense, and those of us who fairly leap into the quicksand of the emergency disciplines can be as career-infatuated as anybody. The rhetoric of disease and cure is, after all, highly seductive. In fact it's downright sexy. That's why so many of us do it.

Dashing from cadaver lab to classroom to library, we surely resembled puppies with our heads out the car window. We were on a mission, teeming with the zeal of the righteous. We would have gleefully run over grandmothers in a crosswalk to get to a good emergency. It's that magnetic.

What bothers me most, looking back, is that I probably had the advantage of more early warning flares than many other fledglings. I could have stepped away before too much emotional and financial investment. We were not even out of med school before recognizing the snollygostery around us. And more exasperating than the misbehavior was the reality that even the most outrageous shenanigans are tolerated within the halls of health care, as long as the outside world continues to be as impressed as we are, by all the good we do.

Those were heady times, for the late 70's had all the trappings of the Renaissance. We were, after all, the pride of our campus – *UCSD School of Medicine* – in the chrysalis of advanced pre-hospital disciplines. There were just not many earthlings doing what we were. EMS textbooks were literally being written by the bright folks who whirled around us each day, and many of our own ideas then are standard protocols now. The books tucked under our arms at the time were physicians' books. Among the first Paramedics in the nation, we were 19 neophytes in lab coats, armed with shiny new stethoscopes, convictions that refused to dwindle and the unmatched energies of troopers on point. You could not have stopped us with a freight train. Some of the best-known newscasters in the country got their start on the same university campus we did. And they often tagged along with cameras to file their rookie news reports on our training adventures, as part of their *UCSD* Visual Arts Program.

We saw ourselves as warriors, prepping for the nobility of battle. We were yet to learn that rescue medicine – at least the rendition practiced on the metropolitan streets of America – was more warlike than anything we could imagine. It was a war where the most deeply wounded were often, strangely, the caregivers. For the cloistered dimension of EMS was rife with 'friendly fire' and grew more so by the year. This of course leads to the logical question of why any normal person would choose the profession. Well, most normal citizens do not. But in our unmitigated zeal to get to the meat of lifesaving, it would have served us well to curb our soaring sense of wonder long enough to notice the enigmas of rescue, for they are in fact appalling. Being of sane mind, we might at least have grown wary of the maelstrom. Hell, we might have turned and fled the other direction.

The sad truth is that in the beginning it is simply not possible for the bewitched intern to fathom the essence of EMS, nor its undercurrents of sheer madness. For these are kept quite deliberately hidden.

So no, I certainly did not start out a skeptic and I would guess that almost nobody does. In my formative years I was as goofily naïve as anybody:

- I stood convinced that health care was fairly insulated from petty infighting so prevalent in less meaningful professions.
- I was certain that saving lives was the highest of its priorities.
- I took for granted that scientific integrity was somehow a given; that there were too many safeguards to allow fraudulent research to harm patients.
- I believed physicians were held to the loftiest of discipline standards.
- I was sure the most prolific drug profiteers on the planet were tucked away in jungle hideouts.

And it was revolting – quite viscerally painful – to concede that not a single one of those beliefs happens to be true.

So what is the purpose of the *Paramedic Heretic?* Simple. It is time for somebody in my field of expertise to shout "gardyloo!" from the belfry. It is time that you – health care's ultimate consumer – gain the perspective of just how distorted our corner of medicine has become. The goal here is entirely uncomplicated. You will almost certainly have need to call 911 for medical help at some point in your life, so you might want to read up, because we just don't think like you do. Before this book is finished you will know exactly how we think, which might come in handy on your next personal emergency.

What you have here is a veteran medic's unvarnished 30-year critique. A professional bloodline; a pilgrimage to heresy. If you are wise beyond your years, you will become a heretic, too. At the very least, when you put this book down you will know – as the marvelous Paul Harvey used to say – "The rest of the story."

Make no mistake. Much of what goes on within the monastic world of medicine is brainsick beyond belief, fashioned in part by some rather ignoble dynamics. For brevity, we call these the *Immutable Laws*. You are not going to learn the Immutable Laws from the network news. You will not absorb them from the internet. If you happen to have medical friends it is unlikely they will fess up, either. In fact, we in EMS don't even admit the Immutable Laws exist.

Until now. Time for the cleansing light of day.

Oh, and one more thing? We always spell Paramedic with a capital 'P'. We think we've earned it.

"A heretic's method of inferential reasoning is simple as soup:
Res ipsa Loquitur"

(The thing itself speaks)
—The Author

"The great enemy of the truth is very often not the lie – deliberate, contrived and dishonest. But the myth – persistent, persuasive, and unrealistic. Belief in myths allows the comfort of opinion without the discomfort of thought."

—John Fitzgerald Kennedy

Introduction

A (Deliberately) Brief History of Emergency Medical Services

How we came to be

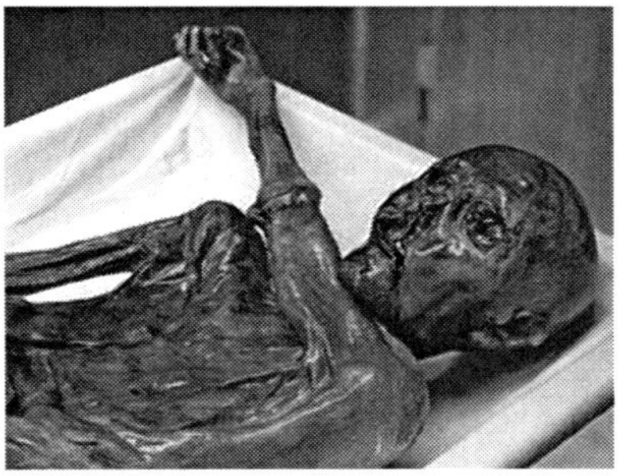

Otzi the "Ice Man" died 5,300 years ago from an arrow wound, in the Oztal Alps, Italy (Photo credit: South Tyrol Museum)

An obscene number of the earliest human remains are unearthed with spearheads in their stomachs and necks and ribs and faces. Along the border of Northern Sudan, for example, lays a fascinating dig site called Cemetery 117 – a mass grave of 59 ancient people. They were men, women and kids and they were murdered 12,000 years ago.

The evolution of what we call EMS is rooted in mankind's predisposition toward slaying one another – or trying to – most notably on the battlefield, but other times in our homes, on the job, on the streets, in the malls, in our schools. It has been argued that humans are opportunistic carnivores, biologically wired to kill, either directly or in the abstract via blood sport. Thus we share a nearly limitless capacity for violence.

The length and breadth of our species' barbarity is arguably the genesis of all first aid. And those not fortunate enough to have a convenient legal war in which to express their ruthlessness, find ample opportunities to draw blood in their very own neighborhoods. This propensity for savagery is not found in every society, but has always been intrinsic to ours. And what this means to you as our new millennium begins, is that when a victim calls 911 for say, a workplace amputation of some fingers, that fingerless fellow can thank heaven for the skill-set of modern Paramedics. Because much of what we do for you and your now detached digits, is the direct result of what we've learned from Viet Nam, the Middle East and good ol' homegrown, inner city blood-letting.

We know that the Greeks employed combinations of wine and oil to treat flesh wounds centuries before the Nazarene walked the earth. They used tourniquets to save hands and feet. We see depictions on ancient Greek pottery of Achilles tending to the wound of a fallen comrade during the Trojan War. We know Roman soldiers improvised sword blades as arm and leg splints during Hannibal's invasion of Italy in the second Punic War. Their 'auxiliaries' employed shields as extrication boards. They cobbled chariots as makeshift ambulances. They were doing all of this and more 2,200 years ago.

In France, Napoleon Bonaparte's personal physician, Dominique Jean Larrey, is credited with fashioning the first known system of field treatment – called then, as now, 'triage.' And this occurred in the late 1790s. The term 'ambulance' itself did not refer to transportation at all until modern times. An 'ambulance' was rather a temporary first aid station – the precursor to the U.S. Army MASH unit. The word 'ambulancia' can be found in the historical writings of Spain's royal family 300 years before that, during the reign of King Ferdinand and Queen Isabella who, as you may recall, funded the expeditions of Christopher Columbus.

In North America 300 years ago, well before we were America at all, our earliest residents learned to fashion a stretcher made of tree limbs and bison leather skins – called a travois – which could be dragged behind a horse to transport the sick and injured to medicine men.

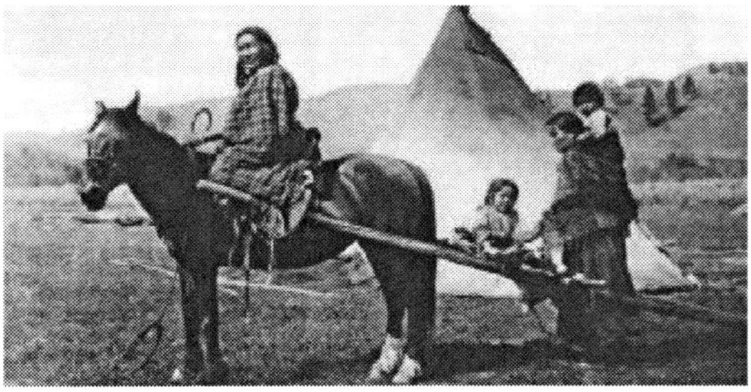

Cheyenne family, horse and travois, circa 1906 (Photo credit: Buzz Tuell)

The first written account of 'mouth-to-mouth resuscitation' – so far as we can tell – happened in Ireland and involved a miner who was found not breathing following the collapse of a coal tunnel, in the 1730s. We have no way of knowing if rescue breathing saved his life. It seldom works today, so the odds are the miner didn't survive either. But a life-saving method was born.

In the United States the first documented application of organized treatment outside hospital walls occurred during the Revolutionary War, when once again the battlefield provided jaw-dropping numbers of injuries, creating the perfect climate for emergent care and transport ingenuity. Leaders of the Continental Army saw need to separate the injured into categories of medical severity, and transport them from small, field aid stations to long-term care facilities. George Washington himself was committed to improving what was, in 1775, an almost non-existent system of organized care of his soldiers.

For the next 85 years the U.S. saw little measurable progress, even though the opportunity to get creative was everywhere. The War of 1812 as well as the Indian Campaign provided trauma that would impress even a modern-day street thug. Alas, few innovations in lifesaving were to be seen. But along came the War of the Rebellion, as the Civil War was known in the North at the time. (It was called the War for Southern Independence in the South.) And first aid found itself once again in dire need of

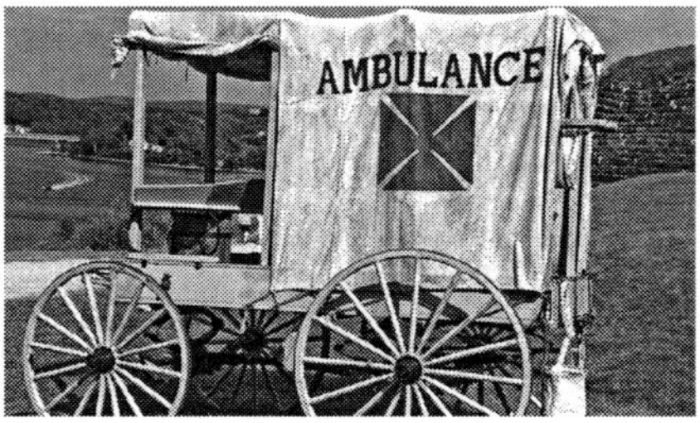

Civil War patient transport, circa 1863 (photo credit: Liz West)

out-of-hospital ingenuity. Deaths due to disarray were appalling. It is significant to note that American physicians were aware by that time that European health care providers were making great strides in emergency management, especially in Scotland and France and Germany and England. But U.S. doctors – as is their wont – steadfastly refused to adopt impressive breakthroughs which were not their own.

On the battlefield crude efforts were made and by war's end, Abraham Lincoln had signed legislation that would ensure at least minimal ambulance service protocols for the military. Non-military folks within growing cities soon took note and civilian ambulance plans came along just after the Civil War, in the mid-1860s. That was when trained hospital staff would jump into carriages that could accommodate patients lying flat on their backs.

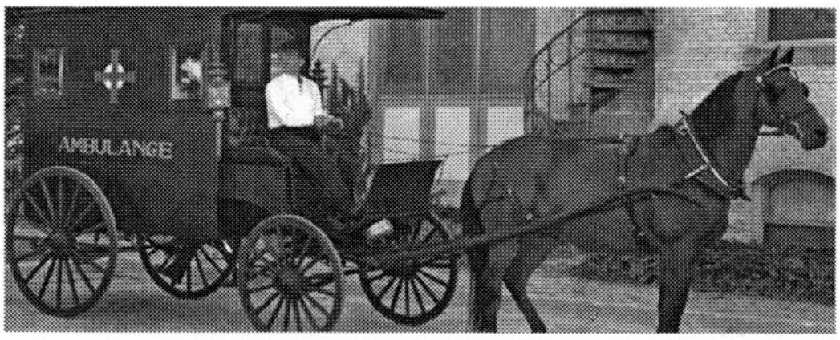

Petrolia ambulance, Ontario Canada, circa 1908 (photo credit: City of Toronto Canada EMS)

Early records can be found in city archives of New York's *Bellevue Hospital* and Cincinnati's *Commercial Hospital and Lunatic Asylum*, as well as a dozen others. But it would still be another 50 years before trained rescue teams were the norm, and even then they were scarce, because they were nearly all staffed by unpaid volunteers. Those well-paid earned a dollar a day.

The most common vehicle for patient transport in the U.S. between the 1930's Depression and the 1960's Cold War, was the mortuary hearse. And more than 12,000 of them cruised city

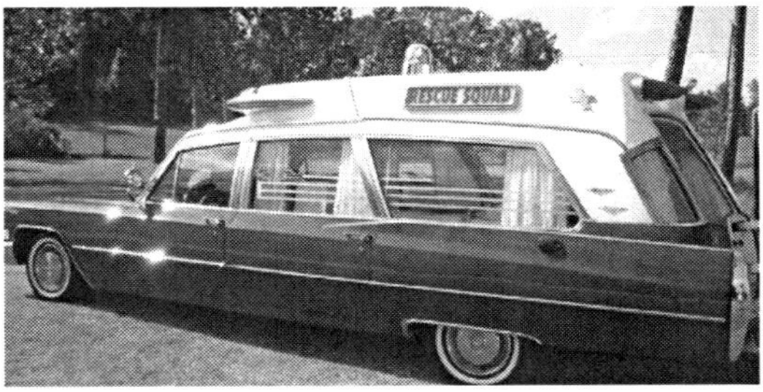

Perhaps the finest of the era was the Cadillac-Superior (Photo credit: Car Pictures.com)

streets during that time. Nearly every town had at least one and they responded by phone on a moment's notice. Nationwide word was spreading among morticians about this nifty new way to make money between funerals. If a decent dollar could be earned handling the dead, outright wealth could be amassed by carrying away the not-quite-dead. They didn't have to fix anybody up – they only had to cart them off. Victims bleeding or not, these 'ambulance attendants' were on an exciting new mission. The guy in the back was a mess but alive! Little wonder their vehicles were called 'meat wagons.' It mattered not at all to the purveyors of this avant-garde cottage industry. They thought they'd won the lottery. How could a funeral home lose? If the customer continued to breathe he or she was whisked off to the hospital and shelled out real dollars. If breathing stopped . . . well, the poor lad or lassie was already lying in a hearse. Either way, somebody paid.

By the early 1960s American physicians were beginning to heed their counterparts in Europe, far ahead of them in nearly every aspect of emergent care. In Belfast they were already operating 'heart emergency' response teams out of hospitals. A full 230 years after the Irish miner was the first known recipient of artificial respiration, U.S. physicians decided that maybe it deserved a closer look. In Baltimore Doctors Peter Safar and James Elam were pioneering a new-fangled chest compression/mouth-to-mouth protocol they believed held promise. In order to teach colleagues how to do it, they joined forces with a Scandinavian toy maker named Asmund Laerdal. Together they designed *Resusci Anne*, a training manikin with an ethereally human face. The face was in fact an eerie replica of a lovely death mask created by French detectives, after finding a young

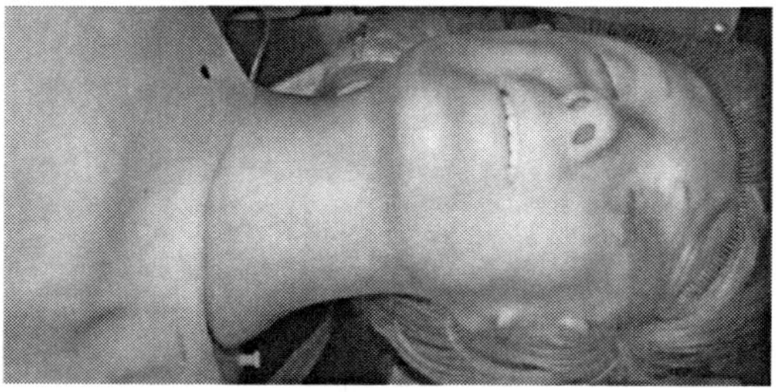

The River Seine girl would never know her future name: Resusci Anne (photo credit: EMS Museum)

girl drowned in the River Seine in Paris, in the 1890s. The gendarmerie never learned her name, but it probably wasn't Anne.

And so it happened that the initial stone of the American EMS foundation was finally laid – the advent of CPR. The realization that rapid intervention could occasionally – but not usually – save lives, triggered the movement toward what we now call Advanced Cardiac Life Support. But there was another aspect of the equation that deserved even more attention.

In the mid-1960s the *National Academy of Sciences* generated a seminal report on the toll that trauma – as opposed to illness – was taking on the citizenry. Entitled *Accidental Death and Disability: the Neglected Disease in Modern Society,* the researchers supporting this paper called the nation's sheer numbers of traumatic injuries an "epidemic" and one of the leading causes of death. Among other revelations the research determined that in nearly all cases, American ambulances were poorly designed; poorly equipped and poorly staffed. Well they were after all, hearses, scarcely designed for anybody with a pulse. They were transporting thousands and saving almost no one. During the Eisenhower era of the late 1950s 3,000 citizens each month expired on streets and highways, and there existed no system at all to quell the growing death toll. Impressive advances in health care were limited to in-hospital and outpatient treatments. Real patient care did not extend to patients crushed in cars. But that all changed the day President John Kennedy pronounced, "Traffic accidents constitute one of the greatest – if not the greatest – public health problem."

Kennedy's speech on street deaths was as much a call to arms for medicine as was his challenge to *NASA* to put a man on the moon. And from that day forward – among politicians and health professionals alike – sudden, collective focus on trauma and coordinated response was born. And none too soon, because a follow-up study revealed that in 1965 alone, vehicle crashes killed more Americans than the Korean War. Evaluating pre-hospital care, the report stated that, "If seriously wounded ... a citizen's chances of survival would be better in the zone of combat than on the average city street."

It bears mentioning, however, that behind the scenes this focus upon – and rapid growth of – pre-hospital modalities, was chafing the comfort levels of thousands of physicians. Basic first aid was morphing into advanced treatment practically overnight and doctors split on whether this was all such a great idea. From "get them into the truck and go" to sending ER talent and stabilizing them first, seemed completely backwards to many. Lots of MDs were still married to the concept that, "fast is good, faster is better." (Indeed, plenty of them still are) And at least some cities where patients were being calmly treated on-scene were also home to EMS' loudest detractors. The naysayers found it difficult to argue with the early innovators like Doctors John Chadborne and Bill Grace, whose Mobile Coronary Care ambulance, operating out of *Saint Vincent Hospital* in New York City, was saving lives on a weekly basis. There was something uncomfortably logical to this odd business of non-doctors treating patients as they lay. But they argued anyway. Ham-strung by lofty opinions of their own intellect, physicians argued with much the same vigor as when they set out to quash midwifery and chiropractors; holistic care and nurse practitioners; acupuncture, chelation and Ayurvedic therapies.

By 1969 non-physician EMS teams were responding to and treating heart patients in pilot programs in Miami, Columbus Ohio, Jacksonville, Los Angeles and Seattle. The *University of Miami Medical School* was one of a handful training a new breed of rescuer, calling them "Paramedics." In Los Angeles, Doctor Walter Graff spearheaded a Mobile Coronary Care Unit with medical teams, which included nurses, responding from *Daniel Freeman* emergency department.

In January, 1970 California State Senator James Wedworth and Assemblyman Larry Townsend introduced a groundbreaking bill known as the *Wedworth-Townsend Paramedic Act.* It was signed into law by Governor Ronald Reagan, which put the stamp of legitimacy on several new roles, most notably that Paramedics would legally perform physician-level care miles away from the nearest physician. Medics would coordinate their efforts via field radio, while communicating with yet another new creature, the Mobile Intensive Care Nurse. EMS was now solidly on the footing of its own specialty, functioning outside the traditional confines of hospital walls, requiring fresh eyes and ears to guide its ever-expanding litany of protocols. Unique and never-tried business models would spawn to manage and finance this new brainchild. The scope of treatment in streets, on mountaintops, in living rooms and worksites, would go far beyond anything envisioned even a few years before. Stratified field caregivers would follow, and carry the ball into the new century.

First Responders:

These professionals are generally firefighters trained in basic first aid, although they are also forest rangers, lifeguards, private security, campground staff and police officers. Their purpose is to stabilize the patient until advanced care arrives. They perform such skills as stopping bleeding; assessing pulse and respirations; administering oxygen; splinting obvious broken bones and using the Automatic External Defibrillator (AED) when a heart stops beating.

Emergency Medical Technicians-Basic:

This level of care extends beyond First Responder capabilities and includes such skills as properly extricating, packaging and moving the injured; spinal immobilization and obtaining basic vital signs.

Emergency Medical Technicians-Intermediate:

The EMT-I is generally considered the highest tier of college-level first aid, allowing the technician to start intravenous lines and administer several medications in the emergent setting. Dextrose therapy for diabetics and adrenaline for severe allergic reactions are commonly given. Equipment such as glucometers for blood-sugar analysis and pulse oximeters for blood oxygen levels are often used. EMT-1 teams transport more than 100,000 non-emergent citizens each day to and from medical facilities.

Paramedics:

Medics are customarily trained to the highest level of advanced treatment in the non-hospital setting, having the advantage of medical school-level education in sophisticated treatments and a thorough comprehension of biological and pathological processes. Paramedics interpret 12-lead EKG rhythm strips; perform endotracheal intubation and needle chest decompressions for collapsed lungs. They deliver babies, defibrillate lethal heart rhythms and administer a range of emergency medications. It is a given in our world that the typical Paramedic is more properly educated and has a better developed pre-hospital skill-set, than the typical physician.

❖

By 1972 millions of federal dollars became available to counties that agreed to adopt the nationally acceptable EMS template. So in cities great and small, highly trained pairs of rescuers started popping up like dandelions on the landscape. But not so fast, Charlie Brown. Not in some cities and certainly not in our city. Not San Diego, one of the largest cities in the nation, a mere 100 miles down the freeway from *Daniel Freeman, Harbor General* and L.A.'s *Emergency* television medics. Our burgeoning border metropolis would wait nearly another decade for the level of street care enjoyed in Podunk, USA.

And why would that be?

In 'America's Finest City' the most vocal opponents of advanced rescue medicine were a handful of MDs who happened to hold pontificating sway over the City Council. They held an equal level of contempt toward these "unproven, unnecessary, probably dangerous" changes. San Diego operated barren police ambulances, and that was quite good enough. The last thing citizens needed was a bunch of pretend-doctors running around in shiny trucks.

So the years went by. Eventually, after nearly a decade of hearing little but a litany of negatives from some of the most respected physicians, the City Council decided to put its collective foot down and vote to approve San Diego's first Paramedic program, to begin in February,1979. Of course an airliner wiping out a neighborhood four months prior, did nothing to strengthen the contrarian physicians' case. The Mayor – and future Governor – Pete Wilson was pushing hard for a true EMS upgrade, and had it not been for his vision and persistence, San Diego might have waited another 10 years. No need to look far for a training program: *UCSD School of Medicine* in La Jolla was, after all, smack in the middle of town, already generating qualified Paramedics for other, more enlightened cities. The highly-intensive curriculum was directed by Doctor Andrew Rauscher, under the School of Anesthesiology. It was overseen by Doctor Silvia Micik. It was managed by Gail Walraven, whose team of instructors were seriously dedicated, marvelous women, everyone: Ginger Murphy. Margie Nerney. Karen LeBlanc. Josie Harding. Marilyn Sheets, who came along just a bit later, should be included too.

Because it was so late in coming we find it noteworthy to reference the first Paramedic-level EMS call in the city of San Diego, which occurred on February 2, 1979, at 8:19 in the morning. The emergency was what is known as a dissecting aortic aneurysm and there exists no condition more deadly. Had this gentleman collapsed the day before, he would have been picked up, loaded into a police van and carted away to die within the hour. But not on this day.

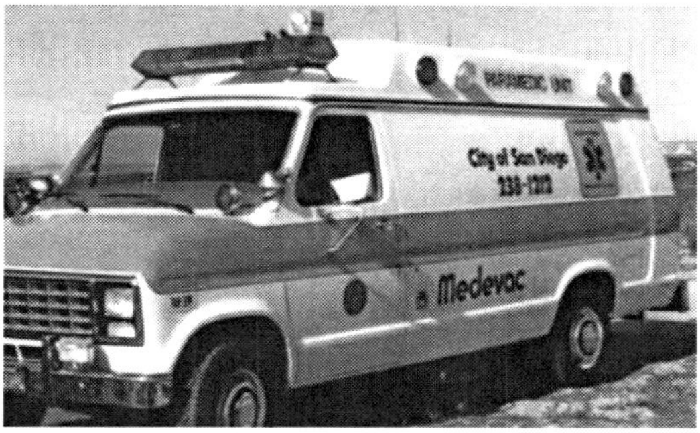

The first advanced EMS units in our city were *Medevac*
(Photo credit: Thom Dick)

The rescue team arrived within five minutes and performed a sophisticated physical assessment. They compared blood pressures on each arm in both sitting and supine positions – a technique likely unheard of by first aiders who came before. They determined a 100% accurate diagnosis. They placed their patient on high-flow oxygen and inserted two large IV lines, running fluid into the man on the kitchen floor as quickly as humanly possible. They interpreted his heart rhythm via a portable EKG monitor called the LifePak 5. They transported the patient slowly, smoothly – red lights but no siren – to *Mercy Hospital.* He was admitted directly to surgery and he lived to tell his grand kids all about his nearly lethal adventure.

Case #7900001 went down in medical history. Mr. Ivan Kosygin, a 66- year-old Ukrainian emigrant. The MICN nurse on the hospital end of the radio was Diana Hunt, with her marvelous British accent. The ER physician of record was Thomas Kravis. The rescuers? Cyndi Stankowski, one of the first women Paramedics in the nation, fresh out of school.

And your author.

"The plain truth is, you're not going to save many lives in your career, and you're setting yourself up for a world of disappointment and disillusionment if that's what you expect."

—Kelly Grayson
Paramedic, Author, "Life, Death and Everything in Between"

Chapter One

Welcome to the Twilight Zone. *Now do us a favor? Go have yourself a truly bad day.*

The day that broke the heart of a city

I had not planned on visiting an airplane crash on my birthday but that's the way this job treats you. You think the biggest part of your afternoon will involve a chocolate cake. Then an airliner comes screaming down into a neighborhood nearby. For a medic, watching the action unfold on television isn't really an option, even on your day off.

So within eight minutes after it happened, by 9:10 in the morning, I was there, walking slowly towards a wall of flames of the worst airline disaster – up till then – in U.S. history. *PSA Flight #182* had collided midair with a tiny Cessna training plane a half-mile above the city of San Diego. And seventeen seconds after the two planes struck each other, the monstrous Boeing 727 exploded into a quiet residential nook, splattering wreckage throughout four city blocks of the neighborhood we call North Park. The impact was literally earth-shaking – powerful enough to register several ticks on the Richter earthquake scale. It took

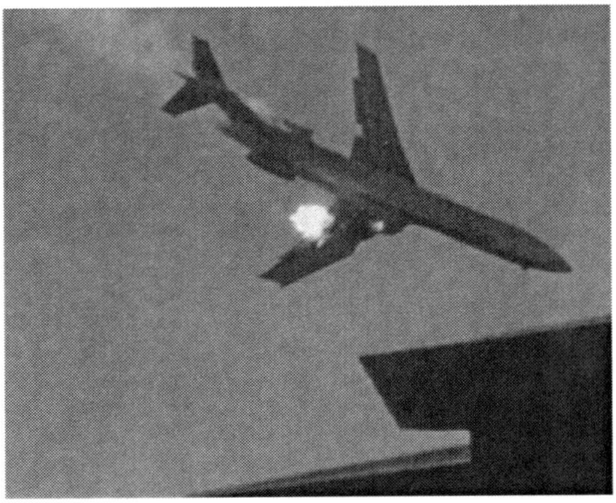

Five seconds before hell on earth (Photographer: Hans Wendt)

the thunder ball all of three seconds to incinerate 22 houses and a dozen cars – as well as trees, front porches, power lines, telephone poles and a playful little pit bull lounging on a lawn.

The human toll was unspeakable: 128 passengers. Seven flight crew. Seven more in homes and cars. Two pilots in the Cessna on a city street not far away. The carnage was – as the *National Transportation Safety Board* determined – the ugly result of three tiny human errors that occurred within a frighteningly brief period of time. Sometimes that's all it takes. A year later, the *NTSB* report would say this:

The causes of the crash were threefold:

- The PSA flight crew did not advise the control tower that they had lost sight of the smaller plane, after initially answering that they had the Cessna in sight
- The pilots of the Cessna failed to maintain their assigned heading, as instructed by the tower
- The ATC controller failed to advise the airliner that the Cessna had veered toward its glide path, even though his warning alert had sounded, telling him the planes were on a collision course

And so it all came to this, and a quiet California neighborhood now resembled your worst vision of ground zero.

At the eastern edge of the impact point I recognized a familiar San Diego police officer, Charles Mattingly, with his arms outstretched, waving off an ever-growing crowd of onlookers. Other cops to his left and right were stringing hundreds of yards of yellow police tape around the entire area. When he saw me he turned and pointed down the street, in the direction of the command post. It was not visible through the smoke and fire, so I walked a wide circle through what was left of incinerated back yards to get to it. The fences were demolished, which made the trek easier. Just down the street, south of the incident command center, a bright orange Coast Guard helicopter squatted in the middle of an intersection – a sight which underscored the already surreal atmosphere. Seven *Hartson* ambulances were assembled, along with a half-dozen Navy units. Nearly all of them would go home unused. After a quick briefing I joined the corpsmen, and for the next two hours we went door to door to every house that was not in flames, looking for injured and calming residents. San Diego's firefighters were everywhere, connecting lines to hydrants, breaking down doors and walls of crumpled homes, in search of survivors. They lifted large sheets of aircraft skin to see what might be underneath. We stayed out of their way as we escorted dozens of crying residents out of the area, to gather at a local high school, until the fires were out and broken power lines shut down.

I recall how we were all in disbelief that day, in that fewer than a dozen people on the ground were hurt, even as hundreds walked in and out of the debris field in a daze. A saving grace was that North Park was a working class neighborhood and most of its residents were – by 9:00 in the morning – already on the job or in school.

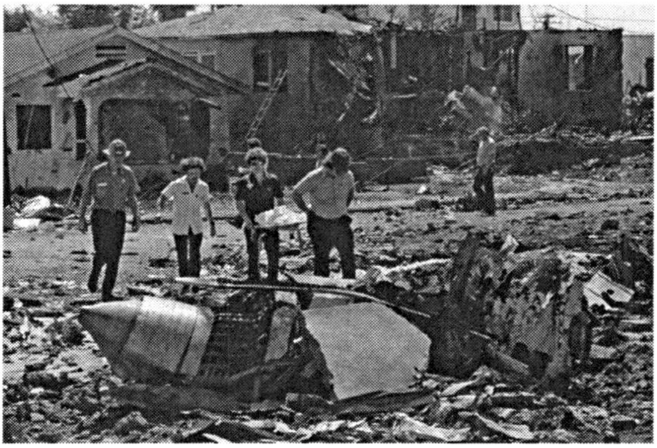

Sadly, there was no one left for us to save (Photo credit: *San Diego Police Academy*)

I circled the tail section of the big plane – known in flight conversation as the 'empennage' – towering above smoldering litter in the street. A single jet engine cowling lay in a heap not far away, its

PSA lettering clearly visible. Well-known *TV39 News* reporter John Britton was there, standing with his back to large flames, speaking into a microphone over the noise. His cameraman battled the heat in his face and kept right on filming.

The stink of aviation fuel in the air was heavy enough to gag us all into submission. *San Diego Police Academy* had brought in a group of cadets to assist in tagging body parts, and they moved through the debris quite slowly, bending and tagging. For some of them, today would be their first and last day of law enforcement. They would leave the program never to return. But at the moment they were tagging the cremated remains of a man and woman who had been killed instantly in their Audi. Their crime had been simply driving down a street when a big plane exploded behind them. They tagged the upper body of a blonde woman on a sidewalk, mid-forties maybe, all but her head and shoulders gone forever. With mouth and eyes wide open, her face was frozen in permanent, tortuous fear. I found it hard to tear my gaze away from the sheer repugnance of what was left of her.

And all the while at each end of the street, TV reporters were gathering to shout our experience all over the world.

One of my strongest memories of that day is how we all kept our eyes glued to the ground as we walked. Streets and yards were littered with what is traditionally considered evidence, and every single bit of wreckage would be collected. But it was almost impossible to avoid stepping on human flesh. The poor men, women and kids aboard this jet had been instantly reduced to countless charred fingers and toes, arms and legs. Splashes of pink tissue and chunks of smoldering torsos were everywhere we looked. Firefighters were absolutely appalled, with no choice but to drive their vehicles right over the top of human remains to get to the hydrants. I recall no more than five complete bodies throughout the neighborhood, and only the blonde woman's face. The medical examiner would collect 10,306 body parts – hundreds on rooftops, thousands so small they could fit into a spoon. In the absence of DNA tracing at that time, all would be buried in a mass grave. The horror of the moment was underscored – as it so often is – by random things: a lower leg with a gold ankle bracelet. A smudged photo of a couple and their daughter. A Mission Beach vacation brochure. A pair of glasses with no damage whatsoever.

But of all the detail etched into the memory loop labeled *PSA Flight #182*, the remnants of the bright pink, flight attendant's blouse hanging from a scorched tree branch truly hurts my heart.

❖

A few final points worth mentioning: there must have been close to 1,000 people in and around the crash scene before the day was over. Law enforcement, of course. Firefighters certainly. Coast Guard, media, bystanders, residents and Navy corpsmen. EMTs from *Hartson* and *Schaefer*. Nurses and doctors had responded and public utility workers shut down power lines. But one particular group of professionals was conspicuously not there: San Diego City Paramedics. Not a single one. The greatest disaster in the city's history? Absolutely. San Diego City medics on scene? Nope.

Why not?

Unapologetic physician codswallop.

The proximate cause of obstacles to progress in rescue has rarely originated with rescuers themselves. The primary barriers to advancement in EMS are cultural. They lay in physician group-think and their outsized sense of importance, for one. It is little more than hyper-inflated lab coat ego. The self-celebration of physician-hood is a jaw-dropping thing to behold, translated into an almost laughable knee-jerk zeal of being the final say in all things medical. In San Diego, a handful of doctors held covert leverage over the City Council, blocking efforts to establish an advanced EMS system. They stood firm with the same fatuous zealotry that enabled MDs in previous eras to keep the microscope from being accepted in the medical sciences for more than 150 years. The microscope, you may recall – like hand-washing and anesthetic surgery – was seen as an insult to the profession and a threat to physician sovereignty. And now, in a nearly inevitable modern-day mimicry, the last thing many physicians cared to see was a barely controllable new species in their midst. These rescue rowdies coming out of schools – if one could believe television news – had the infuriating habit of trampling upon reverent turf called 'doctor.' Unlike nurses, they had the nerve to stand their ground and sometimes even argue a point of contention. Can you imagine? Worse, they ran around outside totally unsupervised.

Worst of all? In some quarters they were being called – Lord help us all – lifesavers. Not even in their nightmares would San Diego's key medical-political players support such nonsense. So they fought it as long as they could. We will not go so far as to say these MDs outright lied to the City Council for 10 years. Rather – in the words of Winston Churchill – we submit they were, "repeated perpetrators of terminological inexactitudes."

You read it here and now you know.

❖

Would you like fries with that shootout?

At 8:45 on a Friday night the best eateries in San Diego were entertaining lively crowds by churning out food by the ton. One of the liveliest, most expensive steak houses around was a place called the Oak Creek Cattle Company, nestled in a nook of woods out on Sweetwater Road. The array of fine sports cars in the parking lot was mute testimony that plenty of folks were willing to spend serious money for a memorable experience. And they would certainly get their money's worth tonight.

As assistant manager Karen Wood would tell detectives later, when the two guys with guns came through the front door she thought it was a prank. But the eyes behind the ski masks scared her, and she was quick to realize this was no joke at all. The dining room of the Oak Creek Cattle Company was long, rather narrow and dimly lit, angling to the right away from the counter and the main doors. At this time of night every table was occupied. The man standing just inside the front door leveled a shotgun at his rapt audience. He announced to the 56 people inside that, "This is a robbery! Don't anybody move! Nobody has to get hurt tonight."

As he spoke the second masked man moved from one table to the next saying very little, making sure that every purse was emptied; every diamond ring, watch and wallet was dropped into a dark bag he held open in front of each table. It was a big bag and quite full, well before he'd reached the last table on his circuit.

The diners – seated in groups of two, four and six, and ranging in ages from 18-74 – were understandably terrified. They could not know what might set these characters into a shooting rampage. So to a person they remained impressively calm.

What the masked men didn't know is that 22-year-old Mike Arrobio, slouched in a booth at the far end of the darkened room, happened to be on a telephone talking to his girlfriend at the time. He leaned down to cover the phone and said, "My God, we're being robbed. Call 911 and tell the cops there's guys with guns in here!"

San Diego County Sheriff investigators estimated later the robbery remained in progress at least six minutes after the 911 call. By the time the fellows in ski masks exited the front door and headed toward their get-away car, the parking lot was nearly surrounded by hidden men in uniform holding some pretty nasty weapons of their own. Just as the pair reached their car – which was, rather humorously, a white Volkswagen Beetle – the police blinded them with a spotlight and announced over a loud speaker, "Stop where you are and drop your weapons now!"

Well, some bad guys actually do that, but these two grew up watching an awful lot of television. Within seconds the scene turned into something that looked for all the world like outrageous, staged theater. One fellow fired off several rounds at a patrol car with his handgun and actually managed to jump into the passenger seat of the VW. Big mistake. It was the very last move he would make in his life. The barrage of gunfire that followed was deafening to the diners, who could not help but peer through the windows of the steak house. Those less curious opted to drop from their seats and dive for cover. The gunfight echoed across the golf course, which ran along the backside of restaurant row. In spite of bullets flying, the other masked man was able to lose himself in the shadows behind the building and into the woods.

The call came into us at 8:57. My partner Dave and I were working a 12-hour night shift out of *Bay General Hospital* in Chula Vista. We were two of eight medics on a mobile intensive care team called *Lifesaver 1.*

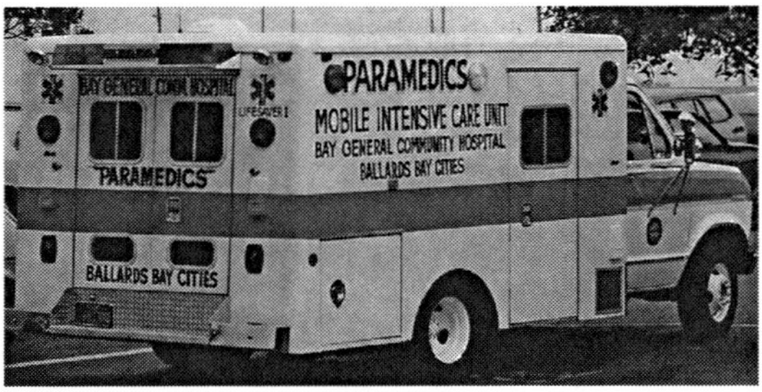

***Lifesaver 1* was unique: a hospital-staffed advanced EMS team (photo: Thom Dick, Paramedic)**

It took us seven minutes to get out there, to the area known as Bonita, and once on scene our driver weaved the Lifesaver unit carefully through the glut of squad cars blocking the street. The first thing that caught my attention was a police helicopter floating out over the golf course, its spotlight searching for the masked man on the loose. The next thing I saw was a male wearing a ski mask, lying on his back in the parking lot, arms outstretched. They had dragged his body out of the car and plopped him hard on the gravel. I went to kneel at his right side, ripped open his shirt and performed a quick EKG paddle check on his bare chest. No heart rhythm at all. He was non-breathing and without pulse. He'd been on the ground nine minutes. I could see bullet holes in his chest, as well as his arms, neck and stomach. The coroner would later count twenty-two in all. I lifted the ski mask carefully and swept my penlight across his pupils. No response. And when I got to my feet I told the cops surrounding me that we would not be working this man up.

"Good," came the answer. Then they handcuffed him.

I walked over to the white Volkswagen to assist my partner. The car looked like a tiny version of Bonnie & Clyde's – bullet holes everywhere. Slumped in the driver's seat was a young blonde female with most of the back of her head gone. Using a gloved hand I pushed the hair away from her face. She was quite pretty, distinctively Slavic, with enough freckles for two or three other women. She was snoring loudly – not entirely uncommon for a massively head-injured patient. Dave told me that he'd found her pupils fixed and dilated, which underscored the fact that she wasn't going to live much longer. We packed the gaping hole in her head with a half-dozen gauze rolls and wrapped it snug. We got her on high-flow oxygen by mask. We slid her limp body out onto a backboard; plugged two large-bore IV lines into her arms, and got her into the ambulance with half the blood in her body pouring out of her head and onto the floor. As long as her heart kept beating, she'd keep bleeding. But you don't put pressure on a class-4 brain hemorrhage.

As our driver was easing us slowly away from the scene Dave peered out the rear window at the line of patrol cars escorting us to the ER.

"Maybe they think she's gonna' wake up and run away?"

I looked out at the red lights flashing behind us, while listening to the heart monitor beep out perfectly regular EKG spikes on the tiny, green screen. They wouldn't be normal for long. It was unlikely she'd even make it to the expensive care unit. I swallowed the acid taste in my mouth. A shootout in a gravel parking lot seemed like a particularly dingy way for a lovely young woman to die. Her face was swelling noticeably and she was rapidly developing two black eyes. Dark red blood dripped steadily from her left ear. I wondered how differently her life might have turned out, had she been a little pickier about choosing her man friends.

I shook my head. "I'm guessing they wish she'd hop out the back door and run down the street," I answered. "They've still got a few bullets left."

❖

Massacre at McDonald's

It was 3:58 in the afternoon on the 18th day of July when a madman calmly walked into a South San Diego McDonald's and opened fire on a room full of diners. For an hour and 19 minutes he continued his rampage. It would finally come to an end when SWAT sniper Officer Charles Foster, positioned on the roof of a post office nearby, stopped the insanity by firing one shot from his high-powered rifle through a gaping hole in the restaurant window.

James Oliver Huberty, a 41-year-old social misfit, would vent his rage at society for more than an hour before his life would come to an abrupt end at 5:17pm. Before our day ended however, we would tag 21 men, women and kids dead as they lay and treat 19 folks with gunshot wounds. And tomorrow we would learn that what we had all just experienced was the single worst civilian massacre in modern U.S. history.

Huberty had chosen his clothing carefully that day: military camouflage pants and a black t-shirt. He armed himself just as carefully: an Uzi semiautomatic rifle; a shotgun and a pistol. The few survivors reported that he said very little before he started shooting them.

"I've already killed thousands. I'm going to kill thousands more."

The first EMS dispatch came out this way:

"Medic 29, Engine 29, a shooting. Details to follow. 522 West San Ysidro Boulevard. The McDonald's. Stage back one block until PD advises further."

One block away, as it turned out, was not nearly far enough. Huberty started firing as soon as he saw the Paramedic unit coming up the street. He was already taking random shots at police and fire units. Once out of their cars, the officers held off returning gunfire because they knew McDonald's had people inside. Our team got there, as did six others, within the next 12 minutes, as well as more than 150 SDPD officers. We all took cover and waited. *UCSD's* new *LifeFlight* helicopter had been dispatched as well, and was landing in a clearing three blocks

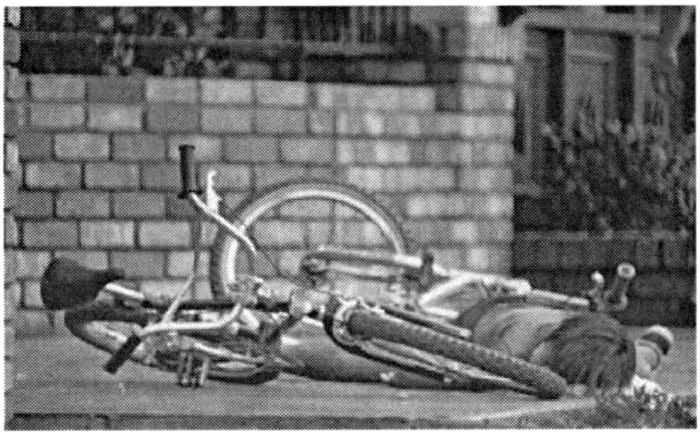

11-year-old Omar Hernandez liked cheeseburgers (Photographed by Barry Fitzsimmons)

away. And within a few minutes we watched 30 SWAT team members surround the restaurant.

From our vantage point we could see three young boys lying on the sidewalk near the doors, their bodies still, their bikes sprawled across their legs. We would discover later that one of the boys – 11-year-old Josh Coleman – was playing dead and would go on to live a relatively normal life. Other people lay bleeding to death in the parking lot. Kids lay moaning in the playground. We all watched helplessly, pinned down by the gunman's bullets.

Police had blocked all traffic along the main boulevard. The downtown area was busy that afternoon, with small shops, a large grocery store and two banks close-by. Huberty would fire off his guns in shorts bursts inside, and then take shots out the windows at anyone who caught his eye. Stores up and down the street were emptied of customers as police ordered business staff to lock their doors and hide away from windows.

The crazed man continued to shoot at everything inside the restaurant: lamps and windows and ovens and walls. No patrons inside could be seen. He was pacing from one side of the dining room to the other, firing shots alternately through holes in the glass and even through the pick-up window.

After the first 20 minutes the shooting slowed, as Huberty now had fewer targets. He would take random shots at pedestrians blocks away and at the occasional cars in distant intersections. During the entire hour I recall fewer than a handful of shots fired in return by law enforcement. Their restraint was impressive. They were all too aware that the tinted glass of McDonald's big windows made seeing any hostages inside impossible.

Then suddenly, from the top of the post office nearby, just above the roof's low wall, a single rifle shot echoed throughout the neighborhood and the massacre was over.

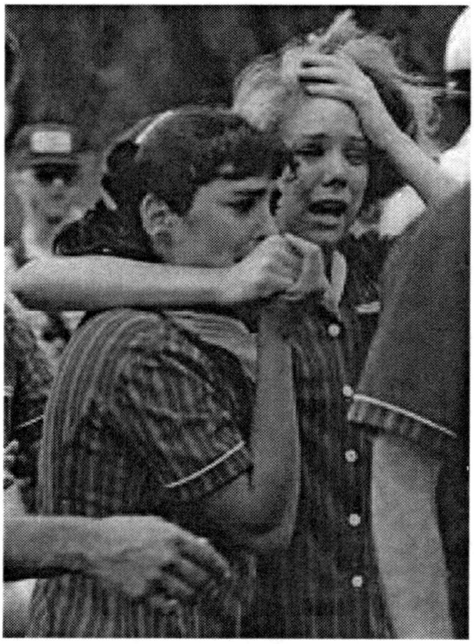

Two fortunate survivors (Photo credit: CBS News)

Six of the SWAT team entered the restaurant first – three at each door – and soon after they were motioning for us. The dread I experienced walking toward that door is almost indescribable. When Huberty first got here the building had 19 diners and six employees inside. We found some of the dead sitting upright in their booths. Some were slumped against the walls. Others lay on the floor, now littered with spent bullet casings. Four of the victims – a family – were aligned on the floor in front of the counter. Sixteen diners and employees were beyond help. Two had French fries in their hands. I checked Huberty personally. He lay handcuffed on the brick floor not far from the North door, with a single gunshot hole in his left chest, just above the heart. His youngest victim was eight months old. The eldest was 74. Over the course of 25 minutes we triaged and treated 10 survivors. Four happened to be staff members who had ducked behind the counter, dashed down the stairs and hidden in the basement. Although understandably terrified, they had no injuries at all. We had six others with gunshot wounds. One was an 11-year-old girl named Aurora. She calmly told us through her damaged face that when the shooting started she crawled on the floor to see if her aunt and the baby were alive. She sensed Huberty standing above her, and "when I looked up at him, he shot me in the mouth."

News media from all over the world were setting up in Southern California for the Olympic Games that year. Within two hours dozens of them converged on the neighborhood of San Ysidro to report on the nightmare. The senseless outrage just made us all so proud to be American hosts to the planet that summer. No one could recall a larger one-day murder toll taken by a single killer. We cleared the scene at 5:34 pm, just as Police Chief Bill Kolender was beginning a press conference in the parking lot. And over the ambulance radio we heard him call the massacre, "Without question, the worst thing that has ever happened in this city and maybe our country."

❖

Two years later my partners and I were summoned to a series of legal hearings. We would sit in rooms filled with lawyers and go over the details of our handwritten incident reports. We answered countless questions. Everything we said was documented by video cameras. Why? Here's why:

In the year after the massacre James Huberty's wife, Etna, had agreed to collaborate with Hollywood producer Lawrence Spivey, hoping to make money by selling movie rights to the story. We were ecstatic when we learned that – as word of the project leaked out – the negative reaction by San Diego citizens was strong enough to stop the movie plan in its tracks. But Etna Huberty just knew there was money to be made somewhere in this once-in-a-lifetime opportunity. So she found an attorney who was enough of a reptile to file a $5,000,000 lawsuit against McDonald's on her behalf. The suit claimed that her husband's shooting rampage was caused by eating chicken McNuggets earlier in the day. Doesn't that make you proud to be an American?

Like the movie and book deal, the suit thankfully went nowhere.

And finally there was this, from the legal summary, the 4th U.S. District Court of Appeal:

"McDonald's cannot be held responsible for the actions of a berserk gunman who killed 21 people and wounded 19 others at the chain's San Ysidro restaurant." In upholding a lower court's finding in a suit on behalf of 26 survivors and victims, the appellate court criticized the corporation for failing to provide even minimal security in a high-crime neighborhood, yet ruled unanimously that, "no precaution McDonald's might have taken would have prevented the July 18, 1984, onslaught by James Oliver Huberty, who was killed by a police sharpshooter."

So now finally, I thought, if we could just keep sociopaths from continuing to breed, folks might not get slaughtered because they decided to go buy hamburgers. And maybe Paramedics would never again see gaping, bloody holes in the chests of dead kids with French fries in their hands.

Too much to ask for?

❖

Question: How many cars can you pile up in a canyon?

It was just after 9:00 on a Friday morning when we got the call.

"Medic 1 . . . a multi-car crash. Southbound Interstate 15 in Cajon Pass."

We stared at the radio and then at each other. We were sitting in the cafeteria at *Desert Hospital* having breakfast because that's what medics do. Now somebody wanted us to waste the best omelettes in Palm Springs. That somebody was very confused. I keyed the radio to give the dispatcher a polite chance to correct her mistake. She certainly didn't mean to call a desert team to a mountaintop 60 miles away.

So I said, "We're en route. Be advised our ETA is approximately one hour."

"Copy that, a 60-minute ETA," she replied, completely unfazed by our outrageous response time. Her tone was a little spooky, which is why I just could not leave it alone.

"You expect we'll find patients when we arrive in an hour?"

"Yes." And then came the clincher. "Be advised 20 units from three counties are also en route."

Twenty ambulances?

Needless to say the trek was a hair out of our normal response zone. Cajon Pass is a sweeping, eight-mile canyon east of Los Angeles that separates high desert communities from the low. From the air it looks like what an ancient asteroid might have done to a mountain range. It holds the distinction of straddling the most active earthquake fault line in North America – the San Andreas. The extraordinary canyon also hosts some of the world's nastiest fog, which is exactly why we were called.

We pulled into the southern, rain-slicked edges of the fog and gathered at a command post. CHP officer John Savage was addressing a news team and we listened in for a moment.

"They had sunlight on the top of the pass and sunlight at the bottom," he said. "This fog bank just blew in within minutes across the traffic lanes. These people had no warning at all."

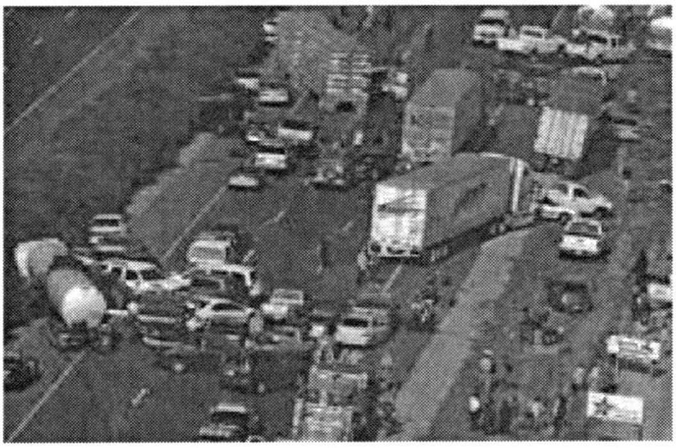

We set personal records that day: 5 hours on scene (Photo credit: Mark Taylor)

One glance up the freeway explained why. The visibility was less than two car lengths. We learned that crews on scene had identified three separate chain-reaction clusters involving 100 vehicles, all in the southbound lanes, a mile below the 4,000 foot summit. Some cars were literally piled atop each other. About 30 were wedged beneath two-dozen tractor-trailers, jackknifed across multiple lanes. The entire scene was a twisted, mile-long junk yard punctuated by crying, moaning, wandering people. There were 52 kids in a school bus too, still sitting in their seats, peering out the windows.

Cal Fire and medics from 12 different agencies – some from as far away as Temecula and Barstow – worked to rescue folks from their cars. Because these extrication teams were already organized, my partner Eric and I were assigned to the makeshift field hospital, set up in a broad grassy area between the northbound and southbound lanes. The grass was tall and wet and a great place to spread out tarps and arrange for bloody folks to lie down in nice, neat rows. A dozen other medics and EMTs moved among them, comforting, tending wounds. And before the day was over we would assess, triage and treat 218 motorists on the big blue tarps, most of them walking wounded. We pinned treatment and transportation codes on their shirts. Every now and then I'd glance down the freeway to the south long enough to appreciate a truly sobering sight: a double line of ambulances, highway patrol cars, Laidlaw buses and tow trucks, as far as you could see.

Over the course of the day we heard various comments among our patients. Here are a few:

"It's real foggy and mom couldn't see anything out the windows," said Deron Knox, age 11, who wasn't hurt at all. "I felt like I was going to die."

"It was just one crash after another, just crash, crash, crash," said Army Specialist Dean Mathews, who was able to crawl out through the broken windshield of his own car. "The most amazing part was that it just kept going on. All I kept hearing was crunch, crunch, crunch."

"One minute it was clear, and the next you couldn't see 20 feet in front of you," said teacher Rey Rodriguez. "Cars were flying all around us."

A big-rig driver with a gash in his forehead was telling an EMT, "I've got to get back to the truck and put a better lock on my trailer. I've got $2,000,000 worth of laptop computers in there."

Jana Ruisch was one of two teachers on the school bus. It was a sixth grade field trip to an airport. "The crash knocked me out of my seat. As soon as I got up off the floor, we were hit from behind by a big truck and I was back on the floor again. Most of the kids are just fine, but we couldn't get them off the bus because the truck was blocking the emergency exit and the front door was jammed."

The car Gene and Bea Hite were riding in was hit four times from behind, which in turn slammed them into other cars.

"It was really scary," Mrs. Hite said. "We saw the fog and stopped, but people just kept driving into it and hitting us. All you could hear were more cars crashing into each another."

Rescue teams told dozens of people to simple remain in their cars until help came for them later in the day. And a lot of good folks did just that, waiting patiently for hours.

Our lone fatality of the day was an elderly woman who had been riding as a passenger in a car. Her heart had stopped before the first medics got to her. There was no way to know whether she had a medical condition or if the trauma of the crash triggered it.

By the time we were packing up to leave it was getting dark. We had been on scene for five hours. We shook hands with *Cal Fire* Battalion Chief Henry Brachais, who made this observation:

"These people were incredibly lucky. This could have been a lot worse."

I looked down at my scribbled notes. One woman dead. Four critical. Twelve serious. Forty-nine taken to hospitals. I took a swipe at the sweat on my face, watching tow trucks haul away more crunched cars. And as we drove home to the desert I could hear a replay in my head of the most prescient line of the day. It came from a nine-year-old brunette rider on the school bus with a broken arm and a black eye. Her name was Alyssa. She'd sat cross-legged on the wet blue tarp, watching the moaning people around her, still clutching a $10 bill in her good hand. She had looked up at me and creased her forehead, mature beyond her years.

"I guess the field trip is over."

❖

The purpose of this chapter is not to boast that my partners and I have experienced some of the most amazing emergencies in history. The purpose is to give you, the reader, a more accurate perspective of EMS than you might otherwise have. We relate these calamities so we can unequivocally state this:

Every rescuer we have ever talked to about *PSA Flight #182*; or the Oak Creek Cattle Company shoot-out; or the 100 car pileup, or the McDonald's massacre, or indeed ten dozen other outrageous calls – every single one of them leaned forward in their seats, eye asparkle. They wanted more detail. They wish to

God they'd been there with us.

So if you, the cogent trier of fact, can recognize that this zeal for experiencing the paroxysm of human crisis runs in the veins of the rescuer, you will be far better prepared to grasp the Immutable Laws. Because they are real; they are unchangeable and the first one is this:

Immutable Law #1
A wretched day in your world is a great day in ours. We happen to love it.

"Is it weird in here, or is it just me?"

—Rod Whyte

Chapter Two

One of us is worth many of you

In our world we call them "compound tragedies." That's when lifesavers become victims themselves. We try to keep them to a minimum.

Historically in some scenarios – those incidents with limited or restricted entrances or exits; sites not designed for continuous occupancy like storage bins, silos, manholes, below-ground fuel tanks, caves, pipelines – more people are killed trying to save others than are killed in the initial incident. The *Occupational Safety and Health Administration* holds studies on lethal, confined-space incidents as an example, showing that when multiple deaths happened, most of those who died were rescuers. The *National Institute for Occupational Safety & Health* has concluded that rescuers account for six out of every ten confined-space fatalities. And that is merely one category.

Chances are, you've heard stories of compound tragedies before. They tend to make the news when they involve electrical lines, mines, floods, traffic crashes and rogue ocean waves.

Sometimes they involve professional first aiders and sometimes they don't:

- Last summer on a Northern California beach, five people in three different incidents drowned in strong ocean currents while trying to save their dogs.
- The year before, near Atlanta, an EMT was killed by a train while trying to extricate a crash victim from a minivan that rolled over onto a railroad track.
- In Rockmart Georgia a Good Samaritan who jumped into swift-moving water to rescue a four-year-old girl he had never met, died from his injuries three weeks after the incident. Michael Patterson, age 43, succumbed to multiple complications as a result of spinal chord damage he sustained when he leaped into the Euharlee Creek to save little Javea Jones. The child survived.
- In Los Angeles two Good Samaritans, both women, were electrocuted within minutes of each other, when they ran to assist the driver of an errant SUV. The driver had rounded a corner at high speed after dark, careened into a fire hydrant and slammed into a power pole. The damaged hydrant spewed water across the lawn where a power line had fallen. Five other people were hospitalized.
- In 2001 in Alabama, 12 rescuers were killed in an explosion while attempting to save an injured miner.

A lot of us believe we would surely rise to the occasion to help someone in a life-threatening situation, no matter how dangerous. And plenty of good folks do. This type of heroism was readily seen after the Boston Marathon bombing, when witnesses rushed toward the explosion to help hundreds of injured bystanders, not knowing if another bomb was about to go off. The scenes of strangers helping strangers are truly heartrending.

But few citizens seem aware that EMS personnel are specifically trained NOT to dash into dangerous situations to save lives. And when we don't, our hesitation literally turns logic on its head, in the eyes of 'normal' people. Except for our mindless penchant for cranking up the lights & sirens at every opportunity (a subject we will discuss in another chapter) we've been taught to not rush at all. We are trained to do exactly the opposite of what the citizenry often hold out as the right thing to do. And the more dangerous the incident, the slower, more deliberately we proceed.

Consider what Nick Schuler, a battalion chief with *Cal Fire*, the largest fire agency in California, has to say.

"When firefighters respond to say, a house fire, the first ones on scene assess the risks of the incident. They perform an outside walk around – shut off the electricity, shut off the gas. If the first ones on scene determine there is a victim inside, they follow a strict 'two in and two out' policy. If two firemen go in, two more firemen need to be available to rescue those."

Otherwise, they don't go in to rescue anybody. Period.

Skilled medics do the same. The more serious the patient – the slower we move. Wasted motion generates more problems. Unfortunately the witnessing public simply does not appreciate a slow-moving Paramedic. In fact, it drives them nuts. Here are a few controversial examples:

Rescue team follows procedure; watches man drown

The water of San Francisco Bay never really warms up. And on Memorial Day 2011, the day 52-year-old Raymond Zack decided to end his life, the surface temperature was 22 degrees above freezing. So once his mind was made up, he simply waded out into the calm surf, stood quite still in water up to his chin and waited for the cold to stop his heart.

This particular drama played itself out at Crown State Beach in Alameda, a city-island tucked into a niche along the Oakland side of the Bay. Like most California beaches there were no lifeguards on duty, and the posted signs clearly stated, "Enter the water at your own risk." There is never a shortage of joggers, bikers and water-sports folks however, so it wasn't long before one of them, Sharon Brunetti, called 911 to report this fellow's very strange behavior. The concerned caller knew that nobody in their right mind stands around in the San Francisco Bay.

The good news that day was that *Alameda City Fire* and police got to the scene post haste. The great news was that they really did feel sorry for the poor fellow and wanted to help. The crappy news was that – like most all other first responders in the U.S. – they operate under strict orders to follow protocol. And the protocol in this case was that Alameda City firefighters did not enter the ocean. They were not – as their policy underscores – lifeguards. So they called the Coast Guard. Unfortunately the Coast Guard boat was far too big to access such shallow water. Worse, their helicopter was busy on another rescue.

Alameda police were in no position to help on a water rescue either. As department spokesman Sean Lynch would emphasize later, "Certainly this was tragic. But police officers are tasked with ensuring safety, and that includes their own safety, when they are sent to try to resolve these kinds of situations. We did not know whether he was violent; whether drugs were involved; whether he had a weapon. We are not ocean water rescuers."

Alameda Fire Chief Mike D'Orazi, for his part, said, "This incident was deeply regrettable. But look at it from our firefighters' perspective. They're standing there wanting to do something, but they are handcuffed by policy."

D'Orazi reminded the press that his department had recently undergone major budget cuts, so his teams had neither the training nor the cold-water gear to go into the ocean safely.

And so – if you can picture the scene – two full fire crews, six police officers, a medic unit and about 45 bystanders all on a beach, watching Raymond Zack shivering offshore, staring back at them. Alameda police estimate Zack stood silent in the water for 55 minutes before he simply fell over and died. An off-duty nurse in a wetsuit, who was also a trained lifeguard, swam out to the man on her surfboard and pulled him to shore. Resuscitation efforts were unsuccessful.

As you might imagine plenty of witnesses were openly critical of – and at times hostile toward – rescue personnel that day. And they made their opinions known when the news cameras showed up:

"Hooray for the civilian with the guts to do something," said Martin L. "This isn't anything new. Last summer I saw cops and fire guys standing on a pier while civilians saved a fellow's life with a jet ski."

"You'd think at some point there would be real concern for him," said witness Gary B. "Those so-called 'rescuers' are a complete fraud."

Another witness, Adam G. said, "This isn't just a problem with funding. It's a problem with the culture, of what's going on in our cities. No one would take the time and help this drowning man."

"Just file this one under, nobody important got hurt. At least all the heroes got to go home. What a bunch of cowards." (Tom R.)

"What has happened to EMS today? Where are the dedicated individuals who were always there before?"
(Erin D.)

"What a sick and depraved society we now are. To have so-called rescuers and bystanders watch as a human being drowns, for whatever reason, is just sick!"
(Angie S.)

"If nothing else, shouldn't the human spirit kick in, at least? At the end of the day, institutions ARE run by people. Rules and regulations. Screw the rules. Just jump in and save the man."
(Keith N.)

Of course, those in the rescue business had a few responses of their own:

Mike H., a San Francisco medic, said, "Call it cold and insensitive, but is it really worth the risk? This man intentionally put himself in danger. How much risk is reasonable for a rescuer without proper equipment?"

Tom A. answered, “As a certified bay and surf rescue swimmer, I could give all of you good reasons why not going into the water was the right decision.”

Mark S. an L.A. medic, added, “Unstable people that want to die. Combine that with untrained responders, equals very bad outcomes for public safety professionals.”

Lee R. Palo Alto firefighter answered this way. “The man didn’t drown accidentally. He was attempting suicide, correct? A suicidal subject goes into the water of his own volition and stays there while fire/police ask him to come back to shore. Say a firefighter goes into the water in a survival suit to the man and gets stabbed. Isn’t this a police situation until he is confirmed to be non-threatening? If EMS responds to a suicidal person they wait for PD to make sure the scene is safe. Does that change just because he is standing in 5 feet of water?”

Lem T., EMT, Hartford Connecticut said, “In my squad we’re plenty brave enough to run into burning buildings or jump in the water. What scares us is going before the review board to explain why we didn’t follow policy.”

Karrie B., EMT chimed in. “Here in Vermont our State Fire Academy actively discourages volunteer firefighters from taking advanced courses like high-angle rope rescue and water rescue. If you’re not trained then you’re not certified. If you’re not certified you’re not a safe part of any team.”

Ken C., a Phoenix firefighter added, “A professional rescuer will be in a position to save many lives over a career. Step outside protocol just because the situation gets emotional, and you’ll have the shortest career in town. Who are you going to save if you don’t have a job?”

Chris M., a medic in Boston said, “I broke protocol once on a tour bus crash. The engine compartment of the bus was on fire and I ran in to pull people out, without putting on my mask. I was very, very lucky to get my job back after a 90-day suspension. The next burning bus I see is just gonna’ have to wait.”

As for the city of Alameda, the final official response regarding this case was this:

"(The) *Alameda Fire Department* does not currently have, and is not certified in, land-based water rescues. The city of Alameda relies on the United States Coast Guard for these types of events."

❖

Firefighter drowns in failed rescue attempt

In the town of Wellington Ohio a firefighter drowned last summer in the swollen Black River recreation area while trying to rescue two stranded teenagers. Investigators now say he should never have gone into the water at all.

Allen "Buzz" Anderson, age 47, a certified swift-water lifeguard, made the decision to enter the river connected to a safety line. But his team could have used an inflatable boat to reach the teenagers, who were at the time clinging to partially submerged trees. This was the determination of James Gorman, an *Ohio Department of Natural Resources* investigator.

A park ranger was eventually able to use another boat to save the teens, who had abandoned their flooded SUV on a submerged road along the river.

Gorman stated in his report that the local fire department did not have an established water rescue plan for the Black River in Wellington Township, 40 miles southwest of Cleveland. The report went on to say that initial rescuers were overconfident in their abilities to handle the current and should not have gone into the water without a plan in place.

"I don't know why the boat rescue wasn't tried first," Gorman wrote in the report. But according to Wellington Fire Chief Bob Walker, the inflatable rescue boat had a motor problem and was not fully functional on the day of the incident.

"That's not an excuse. It's a fact," he said. He has since asked the state to look into the failed rescue so his department can use the findings to improve their procedures.

"We have learned from this tragedy," Chief Walker said.

❖

Nurse follows policy – refuses to give CPR to dying elderly woman

On a bright sunny Tuesday morning in Bakersfield California, 87-year-old Lorraine Bayless collapsed in the dining room of Glenwood Gardens senior living facility and the world grew a little dimmer because of it.

The sadness of the situation got sticky when the nurse in charge called 911, but refused to give the woman CPR when the dispatcher advised her to do so. During the dramatic seven-minute 911 tape released by the *Bakersfield Fire Department*, dispatcher Tracey Halvorson asked the nurse, "Is there anybody else around who's willing to help this lady and not let her die?"

"Not at this time," the nurse replied. She advised the 911 operator that "CPR is against company policy." She did plead for paramedics to come as quickly as possible to help the woman, who had dropped to the floor with no warning and was barely breathing.

Jeff Toomer, the executive director of Glenwood Gardens, extended his sympathy to the family of the woman. But he also defended the nurse in question, because she "followed policy." Toomer reported to the press that, "In the event of a health emergency at this independent living community, our practice is to immediately call EMS for assistance and wait with the individual needing attention until such personnel arrives."

The nurse on the phone, whose first name was Colleen, was asked by the dispatcher if she would, "pass the phone to anyone else in the room – another senior citizen, or a gardener."

Nurse Colleen replied, "I'm sorry. It's against policy and I can't do that."

Paramedics did arrive to treat the woman and transported her to *Mercy Southwest Hospital*, where she was pronounced dead almost immediately.

Bakersfield Fire Battalion Chief Anthony Galagaza stated that the dispatcher, Tracy Halvorson, followed protocol and that fire dispatchers give CPR instructions over the phone many times each year.

Jeff Toomer stressed that his staff also followed policy. "We are not a nursing facility. At Glenwood Gardens, we've found it best to follow protocol."

This case and others like it reveal the gaping disconnect between the way the lay public sees those in the emergency setting, and the way medical professionals actually respond. When the story hit the newswire it generated more than 400,000 internet responses worldwide. Here is a sampling of the differences between public and medical professional viewpoints:

Judi said, "I have never heard of such a ridiculous excuse. If you are licensed it makes NO difference what position you are hired into, you function to the level of your license. To refuse CPR because it's against the policy of the facility makes no sense. If this nurse is either an RN or LVN she should immediately lose her license."

Candice said, "I don't know how a nurse can just sit there and not assist someone when they stop breathing."

Phyllis said, "I work for the health department in South Carolina and I would not work in a facility that had such a rule. A nurse is a nurse and you have a duty to do all you can!"

Mark said, "If somebody is dying in front of me and I can do CPR, I'll do it. The management can fire me if they want to."

Nancy said, "Any RN who would work in a facility that has a policy not to give basic CPR to a patient in need, should rethink why she became a nurse in the first place."

Celia said, "It isn't the staff's decision whether CPR is performed no matter the age of the patient. So CPR should have been done."

Missy said, "OMG! How can everyone there just be okay with the fact that a *nurse* was not doing her job?! I understand that it was against company policy, but don't you become a nurse to save lives???"

Evan LPN said, "If these people are too lazy to do CPR I can only imagine how long it takes to get a bath at that place."

Markus R. said, "It's a residence for the elderly. So you already know people are going to be sick and need help, but you set policy to *not* help?"

Joe P. said, "This nurse is a disgusting example of a human being and her license needs to be revoked ASAP. What kind of person who is trained on how to save lives, stands there and lets someone slowly die in front of them and attempts to use some nonsense policy as an excuse. What a disgusting person."

Here, on the other hand, are a few comments by EMS-types:

Michael N. said, "I work at a senior living – not a nursing – facility, and trust me. We are absolutely not allowed to perform CPR. Rules are rules."

Devon S. RN said, "Doing CPR on an 87 year old woman in cardiopulmonary arrest who probably had other co-morbidities is, in my opinion, not in the patient's or the family's best interest. A lot of CPR is, in the end, harmful."

Tammie N. said, "As hard as it is to listen to the 911 call, the nurse did the right thing. The patient had signed a 'Do Not Resuscitate' instruction and her wishes were respected. The daughter of the patient supported the nurse not performing CPR. The nurse was professional and followed the correct procedure in an extremely difficult situation. I hope the staff I have when I am 87 also respect my wishes and act accordingly, even if they personally disagree."

Eppy S. said, "A very unfortunate situation. She was only doing what she was trained to do. Like others have said the woman could have had end-of-life wishes to not be resuscitated. To do CPR on someone who is 87 is cruel in my opinion. Every rib breaks. For some reason in America we feel like death is not an option. Well, it is a natural part of life and it will happen to all of us."

Eric S, Paramedic said, "This ain't television folks. CPR almost never works, especially on an 87-year-old. And there's a real good chance the patients and the nurses have already talked. Maybe the lady had already told them she didn't want it performed on her when the time comes."

Benni BSN said, "Many elderly do not want hard-core resuscitation done on them for various reasons (chronic illness, religion). They just don't want their last days or weeks to end that way. Who knows what this patient might have already told the nurse?"

Babs the Nurse said, "There was no information in the original story addressing whether this woman had given instructions that she did not want CPR. This is very commonly requested by people in their later years. This news reporter may be more intent on sensationalism than factual reporting, it seems to me."

Lindy EMT said, "The point here is not that an elderly woman died. The point is that a woman trained in CPR refused to do it, and why. What this article does is highlight how some health care policies look, to people on the outside of the industry. And you have to admit some of our protocols seem pretty insane to 'normal' people."

And finally, Lisa A. said, "I think that the sad part of all of this is ignorance. People do not realize the process of DNR and no CPR, per patient or family request. I am a nurse. I have done CPR on elderly patients. I have felt the ribs break beneath my fingers. My thoughts were of the pain I was causing the dying patient. I wondered if the lungs or spleen were punctured. What are they thinking in the last seconds of life? Their grimaces told the tale. I have also been with dying persons, and watched them die peacefully while I held their hands and spoke softly into their ear, with peaceful looks on their dying faces. Allowing someone to die the way they want is not evil, wrong or disgraceful. It is a loving gift, their last gift. Please understand that nurses advocate, try to heal, protect and care for people. We love our patients enough to let them die in peace."

Lorraine Bayless' adult daughter agreed. She told television reporters that she was satisfied with the retirement home's protocol. She did not want CPR performed on her mother. The daughter is herself a nurse.

❖

This particular case happened in England. It could have happened here and probably has:

Paramedics refuse to jump into canal to save dying motorist

When 30-year-old Michael Thornton skidded his Land Rover into a channel of muddy water, his truck flipped over on its top and he was knocked immediately unconscious.

When the ambulance team arrived on scene they performed a quick 'risk assessment' and decided it was too dangerous for them to enter the ditch.

In the week that followed an irate medical examiner loudly criticized the medics who – as they documented in their field report – "held off going into the water because we did not want to breach health and safety rules."

A police officer arrived on scene and immediately jumped into the canal – where the water was about five feet deep – and pulled the victim to the grass. The medics began CPR but were unable to revive him.

Coroner Michael Rose addressed the news media when he learned the details of the event. He said the tragedy was proof that England was becoming a nation of cowards.

"I will not say what I think of health and safety regulations those men operate under," he said. "But I was brought up in a country where men risked their own lives to save the lives of others. That was a period in our history which has almost ceased."

The Somerset coroner went on to say, "I do praise the actions of the police officer." He declared the death was "Accidental," that victim Thornton drowned with complications of a head injury and alcohol.

South Western Ambulance Trust said its staff had "made the right choices" and had given the "best possible care" to Mr. Thornton. A spokesperson said, "The Trust is confident our medics made an appropriate risk assessment on arrival at the scene and administered the best possible care in what were particularly difficult circumstances. Paramedics often have to make critical decisions in the most challenging of circumstances in order to maximize the chances of survival for patients.

"There is no question that during this incident the medics made exactly the right choices and performed admirably. They followed the rules."

❖

Man falls through the ice while rescuers make a plan

In Champaign Illinois last winter 20-year-old Kenneth Brown drowned after falling through the icy surface of a small pond. Brown, who had been the subject of multiple 911 calls all day because of loud, disruptive behavior in local stores, was seen running across a grocery store parking lot away from police, who had pulled up yet again to question him about his continued outbursts. But he decided to jog away, directly onto a frozen pond. In less than a minute on the ice, he fell through.

The first rescue team arrived within five minutes and was soon joined by two dozen more firefighters. The man in the water was struggling to hang onto the edges of the ice. According to Deputy Fire Chief Eric Mitchell, "we have several different positions that have to be filled to do a water rescue safely. We have people assisting other people into dry suits. We tether everybody together. We set up a perimeter around the victim on the shoreline."

Mitchell went on to explain that for every rescuer who might end up in the water, there is a support person manning a rope attached to them. And for every rescuer about to go in the water, another is suited up just in case something goes wrong. And while all of this is going on, others are tossing rescuer rings and trying to get the victim to grab them, while still others are inflating a rescue raft. All of this, he said, takes an agonizing amount of time.

"We follow rescue guidelines," Mitchell stressed. "This isn't a safe situation for anybody. Of course I could hear bystanders yelling at us to 'hurry up.' People screaming that we were 'fiddling around.' Our operation might look like fiddling around while a man drowns, but believe me, it isn't."

Later, to the news media, Mitchell explained further. "We're making sure every person on the team is safe to do the job. We are not about to lose a rescuer just for the sake of 'hurry up.' That isn't smart."

Here are a few responses to this story from people in the business of rescue:

SillySafetyGirl said, "And those rescuers are all still alive to respond to calls today and save other lives. I'll take an alive rescuer over an alive civilian any day."

Maverick Medic Manny said, "I remember the time, back when I was young and full of myself, I probably would have jumped right in with a rope in my hand. I've since learned that if you pull a Rescue Randy act out there, you're risking the lives of your team members. Do that and you deserve to get your butt fired."

Anonymous EMT says, "Only fully prepared personnel should enter dangerous water. With no PFD or wetsuit on, you only risk becoming a victim yourself. Then who is going to attempt a multiple rescue? Now you have two victims and maybe three or four."

Paramedic Adam said, "If I step outside those protocols, no matter the outcome, I'll get stomped on and fired, no questions asked. Then I'm no good to anybody."

Fire captain Mark said, "Absolutely I am going to defend the actions of public safety workers who made a calculated risk assessment and didn't go in the water until they were ready. That's why we have protocols in the first place."

❖

Paramedics allow school principal to block ambulance access to injured football player

In San Jose California a high school principal was under fire last year as the result of following a 'no ambulance on the field' school policy. Fourteen-year-old Keanu Gallardo had suffered a concussion during a Del Mar High School football game in October. But even after the *American Medical Response* ambulance arrived, the young player was forced to lay and wait for the medics to haul emergency gear nearly the length of the field.

Then he had to be carried the same distance back to the ambulance.

Del Mar Principal Liz Seabury told reporters she was following district orders which forbid motorized vehicles on the newly remodeled field.

Days later as the young man was recovering, the incident continued to infuriate a number of local town-folks who stated they simply could not fathom a policy that would place turf value over an athlete's welfare.

Parent Debbie Musquez, who witnessed the event, said, "The child's health needs to come first. The behavior of the principal and medics is disturbing."

Campbell Union High School District board member Matthew Dean saw the incident this way. "It's a failure to apply common sense across the board."

The father of another player said, "The principal should have made a different decision. But the *AMR* medics should certainly have overridden her. They knew he had a head injury – they were told as much on dispatch. The medics are supposed to be the 'experts' and yet they let this non-medical professional dictate emergency procedure. That's crazy."

Another parent said, "What kind of environment have we created, such that three adults don't feel comfortable overriding a rule?" he asked.

While it is now clear the delay had no negative impact on the student's health, EMS professionals agree that when a player has a head injury, there is no immediate way to know how serious it may be, so no delay is acceptable. The school district superintendent has since responded with an apology to the injured player's mother. And the district-wide policy has been reversed, to allow access to emergency vehicles if paramedics deem it necessary.

AMR, on the other hand, anticipates no change in protocols at all. The company's policy is – and has always been – that Paramedics do not challenge anyone of authority on scene, regardless of whether such assertiveness may be in the best interest of the patient.

❖

Tragedy in Palm Springs

I had not planned on a Girl Scout bus careening off a mountain road two miles away, but that's the way this job pokes you in the eye. One minute you're lazing around a swimming pool on your day off, gazing at lightning in the distance. Minutes later you witness Sonny Bono act like a chimp on chocolate at a deadly crash site. It was 3:36 in the afternoon when the phone rang.

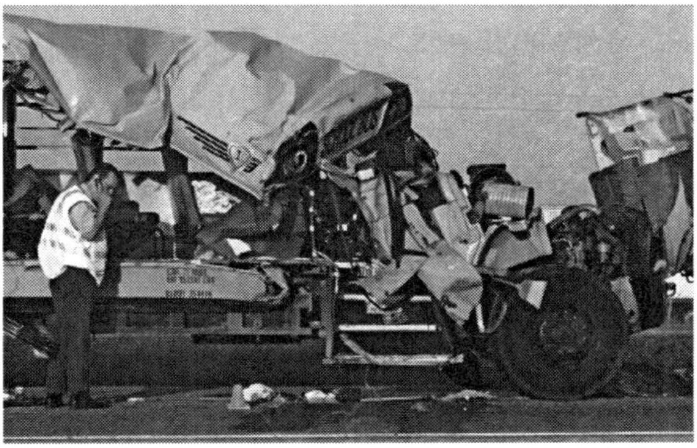

(Photo: Riverside Press Enterprise)

Riverside County Fire communications reached me at home because somebody remembered I happened to live across the street from Tramway Road, out at the extreme north end of town. The nearest medic teams – which I supervised – were scattered across 12 desert cities and would take a while to get there. Tramway Road is a winding ribbon of asphalt; an unrelenting 7% grade rising high into a niche in the San Jacinto Mountains. It dead-ends at Valley Station, the takeoff point for one of the more spectacular cable car rides on earth. Earlier in the day a caravan of traveling teenagers had thrilled to their two-mile adventure up and down the summit. But on the ride back to town an unspeakable tragedy struck. Unfortunately, one of the drivers was a 23-year-old with absolutely no mountain experience whatsoever. So trying desperately to descend a steep grade in third gear of a school bus with poor brakes, was the last mistake he would ever make.

My car jerked to a halt behind the first squad car on scene, with Officer Ralph Landry skidding to a stop right behind me. The crumpled bus was easy to see, off to the left at the bottom of the rocky hill, about 150 feet away. Tourists coming down the mountain were stopping to gather in the middle of the road, staring at the crash site. Because flashfloods have a tendency to wipe out desert roadways, the pavement is elevated about 10 feet above the sandy slope. The big bus lay on its left side with the rooftop towards us. Long, arching skid marks were visible as far up the road as we could see. From the gouges at the edge of the road it was clear the huge vehicle had flipped to its right as it left the pavement, then continued to roll over until it slammed to a stop against the largest boulder on the slope. So nasty was the impact that the body of the bus was torn away from the chassis. But to me, nothing about the scene – not even the bleeding, weeping girls making their way up towards us – was uglier than dozens of head-shaped dents running the entire length of the roof.

One of the most misunderstood aspects of EMS is multiple patient protocol. The first rescuer on a scene does not treat anybody, no matter how badly hurt; no matter how sadly you feel. In truth, we are meagerly prepared for empathy, so this usually works. We are, rather, highly prepared for skills performance. Relating to damaged creatures of our own species in any humane way is neither taught nor demanded. In fact, it is frowned upon. Too often – like so many physicians – medics choose to ignore the fact that laying a momentary hand on a stranger in comfort often makes all the difference.

So poor 15-year-old Debbie had an obviously fractured skull and was barely conscious, draped across a large boulder. In our world it would be an unforgiveable error of the amateur to stop and help her, with a dozen others scattered about. In this case, we had 55. So I stepped over her and kept walking. At this stage in my dementia, 15 years into the business, my poverty of sympathy was well-established.

The priority is to manage the scene, which you cannot do until you know the size and scope of the problem. I could hear an officer on a radio calling for, "all the help we can get" so I made my way carefully down the rocky slope, passing more wounded girls along the way. A detective in plain clothes next to me was doing the same. The scrub brush and crevasses looked like rattlesnake heaven and the footing was awful. We climbed down to the front of the bus, which had taken the brunt of the impact. The driver lay dead across the dashboard. We checked him briefly and then peered through the destroyed front end of the wreckage. All of the windows had been destroyed. At the far end of the bus at the rear door several teenage girls were crawling out. Between them and me lay at least three dozen young women. They were contorted along the left interior wall, moaning, crying, dying.

I used my radio to advise dispatch. "We have at least 50 young women who need immediate attention. We have one adult male and at least 3 females 1144."

Scattered around the wreckage were hundreds of personal belongings. New running shoes and vacation T-shirts. Sports bags, picnic coolers, bright yellow Girl Scout scarves. Sunglasses and wallets seemed to be everywhere.

Inside the grotesquely twisted bus we nearly suffocated in the desert heat. Over the course of about 40 minutes Doctor Dan Cosgrove from *Desert Hospital*, another physician and I assessed those who were not breathing; covered their faces as dead, and moved on to the next. Two of the bodies were lying on top of victims still alive. It was a challenge moving the dead girls aside. Around us men were using extrication boards and Stokes baskets to lift the surviving teens and their chaperones out of the wreckage and up to the pavement, which would serve as a triage area. Paramedic Mike Allison and his partner pulled up. Other medics, EMTs, firefighters and hospital staff were arriving too, tending to some pretty hideous wounds up there. City PD Sergeant Ron Starrs was on scene, bringing a level of order to the chaos. Because it was the last day of July the road surface was extremely hot, so the street was covered with sheets so the injured could at least lie down. We divided our patients by severity of injury, with the unconscious head-injured first to be sent off. Later we would realize that every item of splints, bandages, towels, bed sheets; and IV fluids that nine ambulances had to offer was used up.

We overcame numerous challenges that day, but none more frustrating than the appallingly simple matter of the narrow street. Tramway Road is no more than 25 feet wide with no shoulder at all. The pavement sits atop a berm of boulders 10 feet high, four miles long. By the time we were ready to start transporting patients the entire road was cluttered with dozens of patrol cars and ambulances, fire apparatus and tourists. We had no way to turn around.

At some point in an amazing stroke of good fortune, a private helicopter landed in the sand on the opposite side of the road. The pilot came jogging over to ask if he could help. I said "absolutely" and over the course of the next two hours, his marvelous aircraft shuttled trauma patients down the hill and out over treetops to different hospitals. As the scene began to clear we found we had enough room to finally get ambulances turned around, and somebody was clever enough to suggest calling taxis for the walking wounded. Thanks to creative transportation, we were able to send 19 of the girls as far away as John *F. Kennedy Hospital* in Indio and a few to *Eisenhower Memorial* in Rancho Mirage. This allowed *Desert Hospital's* trauma team to focus on their 21 patients, at least seven of whom were critical. The dead on scene were three teenagers; two chaperones and the bus driver. And later that night one of the girls with a critical head injury died in surgery.

It is interesting to note that at one point I realized Mayor Sonny Bono was kneeling beside me in the sand, supporting a young woman's arm as I placed an IV into her vein. Through broken teeth she was telling us her name was Shelly. She said she was 17 and lived in Maryland. She told us she was one of the lucky ones, getting to go on the California Dreamin' tour. Mayor Bono's face twisted in anguish. I showed him how to hold the pressure dressing on her forehead, which was split open to the skull and bleeding into her eyes. He was clearly horrified at the blood running between his fingers. Later, as the day wore on, I got glimpses of the Mayor hopping nervously between patients as they lay in a long row on sheets in the street. He would hold their hands and touch their faces and tell them they were going to be fine. And in all the commotion of the afternoon, I could not help but notice that Sonny Bono was crying as hard as any of the bleeding girls around us.

❖

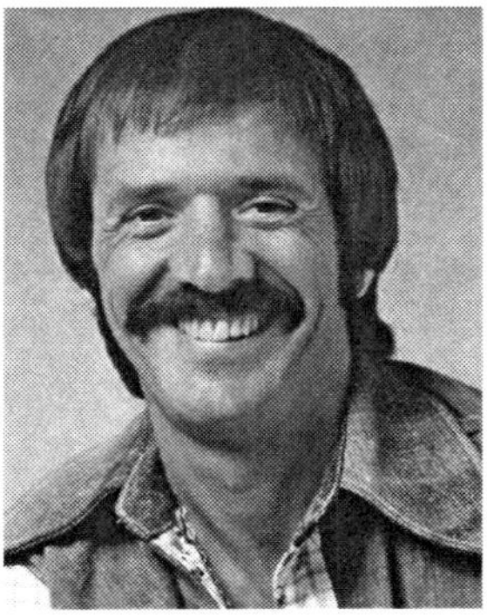

Mayor Sonny Bono (Photo: P. Springs City Hall)

It was a few weeks later when I found myself sitting at a table, amazingly, having a quiet lunch with the famous Sonny Bono. No need for reservations – it was his restaurant. It was also his idea. The layout of Bono's was extraordinary enough to mention, with world-class tennis courts on each side of the building and plenty of windows to watch the action. The courts were flawless green and set lower than the landscape, providing a bird's-eye view from the tables inside. That was no accident, either. Sonny wanted his celebrity friends to feel comfortable, without the annoyance of the desert wind. And he knew very well that paying customers would flock to a place where they could watch people as famous as he was, running around in shorts. I couldn't help but notice some of the shorts myself. Johnny Carson was out there, engaged in a serious match with somebody, and Stefanie Powers sat with elegant ankles crossed, sipping something cold under an umbrella. Her television show, *Hart to Hart,* came immediately to mind. I smiled to myself. On some days the village of Palm Springs can honestly bumfuzzle the brain.

Inside, the penne pasta was delicious. Mayor Bono had listened to my opening spiel and now he sat with his fork suspended above his plate, staring at me in rapt attention. The expression on his face was one of utter shock.

"Are you honestly saying that this county – *our* county – is deranged enough to pull your Paramedic license because we used that helicopter?"

"Not the whole county," I answered. "Just the EMS part."

"How can anybody be that pea-brained?"

I shrugged. "The helicopter was not EMS-certified. Not the aircraft, not the pilot. They were never approved to transport patients."

He plunked his fork down and screwed up his face as if the whole world had gone mad. "That helicopter was a godsend out there. It was like . . . divine intervention! What kind of fools would let those girls lay out there in pain a minute longer than they had to?"

"The kind of fools who don't like medics making independent decisions."

"So what about the taxis?" he said. "I suppose we shouldn't have used them, either."

I sighed. "To tell you the truth, I'm surprised they didn't make that an issue, too."

He groaned. "There's something wrong in the heads of people who think like this. They were probably normal till they got a little authority."

I toyed with my iced tea. "I had about 30 seconds out there to make a decision. It made perfect sense. You saw the traffic mess. I made eye contact with the battalion chief who was busy on his radio at the time. We pointed to the chopper and we both nodded. He agreed, but it was my call. I don't know that he even had time to talk to the pilot. That puts my certification on the line."

He shook his head. "Sometimes I'm ashamed to call myself an American."

My sentiment exactly. I swallowed some food and spoke quietly. "Mr. Bono, you're a decent man. You were the most humane person out there. It took me a week to realize that. And because of that decency, you'll probably never understand what I'm going to say next." I paused to stress my point. "For all the good it does, rescue does not exalt moral courage at all. To the contrary, it squelches fortitude almost by reflex. In the world of EMS, saving lives is *not* the priority. Following every rule every-time, is the priority. You get creative; try too hard to save people? That's the fast track to a short career."

Sonny cringed as though in pain and I suspect he probably was. His rock star days were behind him now. He was a normal person these days and this peek into the *Twilight Zone* was like a kick to the stomach.

He said, "Do you know why I became Mayor of Palm Springs?"

"Not really, no," I replied.

"I ran for office because some small-minded bureaucratic twits wouldn't let me put a sign up for this restaurant."

"Wow. So instead of fighting city hall, you became city hall."

"Sometimes you've just got to out-sneak the bastards."

I nodded. "Well, you certainly have a great sign out there now."

We sat silent for a time as we finished our lunch, but when he spoke again his voice grew lower, calmer, filled with resolve. There was none of the high-pitched nervousness that seemed his norm. I realized there was more to this man than being Cher's former husband, or the overly emotional fellow in the presence of dying teenagers. Sonny Bono had not gotten where he was by dodging challenges.

He leaned forward in his seat and narrowed his eyes. "I have an idea that might work. By God, they are *not* taking away your Paramedic license."

❖

A peculiar thing happened not long after that conversation. Truly curious. A newly minted organization called the *National Disaster Conference* suddenly convened at the Palm Springs Convention Center with surprisingly little lead time. Nobody in EMS had even heard of them. They chose their first-ever meeting to discuss the bus crash at length and to honor Mayor Bono for responding personally and aiding the young victims. They read the names of rescuers, firefighters, police officers and the three doctors on the scene. They thanked the hospitals and the Radisson Hotel, which housed victims' families free of charge. And they ended the ceremony by having the helicopter pilot introduced on stage. Lastly, they asked me to come out of the audience to stand beside the pilot, and the master of ceremonies thanked us personally for our, "lifesaving interventions on your days off." He called us heroes. We all received a standing ovation, carried by the three local television news teams in Palm Springs, as well as *Eyewitness News* from Los Angeles.

I was dumbfounded.

Two weeks later my head spun yet again – this time by a formal letter from *Riverside County Health Department*, advising me that, "Upon further review" they saw no need to proceed in the matter of a "Paramedic breaking field protocol on an unprecedented, extremely challenging multi-casualty incident." So the case of the unwanted helicopter was officially closed.

Back home at the swimming pool I'd come full karmic circle. My one bedroom condo faced the mountain, so I lounged on a lawn chair and gazed up at Tramway Road, weaving its deceptive path through the canyon where the ghosts of Girl Scouts now lived. I thought about Sonny Bono and his "idea that might work" – the totally mysterious *National Disaster Conference* which flew into town and then flew out. Unbelievable. Who in the hell *were* those people? I shook my head with a smile, recalling some of the last words he said to me:

"Sometimes you've just got to out-sneak the bastards."

Well Sonny, I cannot fathom how you did it, but you certainly pulled it off. And Lord rest your soul, I owe you one.

❖

At one point during our lunch Sonny Bono had asked, "So in other words, we've reached a point where a rescuer can't say 'screw the rules' and just do the right thing?"

Not in other words, Sonny. Those are the perfect words.

Immutable Law #2

Saving lives is not our priority. Following our policies is our priority. Protecting ourselves comes next. Avoiding lawsuits comes third. You come somewhere after that.

"When you enter med school you get a ticket to the freak show. When you graduate you get a front-row seat."

—Les Miller MD
Once known as 'Surgeon to the Stars'

Chapter Three

Okay, tell us again. Nurses want to marry . . . whom?

Time to lighten the mood by stepping away from tragedy and here's a subject that just might do the trick. Trust us, during medic down-time this topic is a real thigh-slapper. Let's start this way:

In my formative years – had the subject come up – I might have opined that sure, some nurses probably do lean toward that career in order to marry physicians. But the *Immutable Laws* have a way of spinning your head toward true North, and they certainly educated me on this one. Over the past 30 years we have had ample opportunity to learn the truth, but just to ensure that our own conversations with nurses were not entirely skewed, we put the following question out to LVNs, RNs, MICNs and MSNs in all 50 states. That's several tons of "N's." Just under 600 responses came back. In no particular order at all, here is the exact question, and a representative sampling of their answers, word for word:

“Have you or anyone you know, become a nurse in order to marry a doctor?”

Well, tighten your seatbelt because here come their responses:

“How very stereotypical of you to assume it is a nurse’s ‘fairytale dream’ to marry a doctor. I myself am happily married to a firefighter.”
(RN in May)

“I’m engaged to a med student. I knew him before he ever got accepted to med school. But I’d marry him even if he was a garbage collector. I have lots of friends who are in med school and they do not look down on nurses in the least. I think it is the older doctors who disrespect nurses so much. Hopefully the attitudes of the younger ones won’t change for the worse.”
(Emerald)

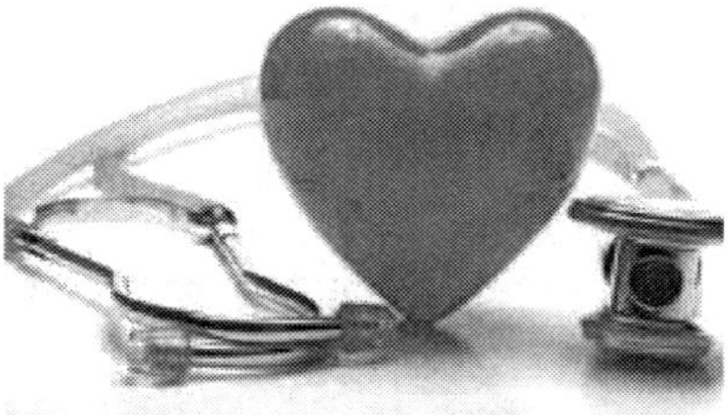

“Not married to one but dated a few. I work with radiologists now and they tend to be impossible. They expect perfection in absolutely everything in their lives. Some of their qualities don’t translate into happy relationships. Many are on their fourth marriages. I haven’t met the doctor yet that I would want to be in a long-term relationship with. I married a teacher.”
(Julie)

“Some of my friends asked why there is so much doctor-bashing by nurses. That’s easy. It’s because nurses get bashed so much by doctors. Their holier-than-thou attitudes don’t make for pleasant comments.”
(LasVegasRN)

“Years ago I had a friend whose greatest desire was to be the third wife of a particular Jewish neurosurgeon. Her theory was that the third wife will inherit everything and in the meantime she could cope with pretty much any negative part of the relationship. Her theory ended when she realized he refused to take his shoes, socks and beanie off when they were naked in bed. She married a teacher instead."

(Gomer)

"The last time I slept with a doctor I was eight years old and afraid of a thunderstorm. Yes, I was a doctor's kid. I once believed there was very little difference between God and my father. Now I would love to grab him out of the grave just to let him know what I've grown up to think of these freaks. After working at a level-1 trauma center, these guys have really lost their luster. I have to agree with most every nurse I've ever talked to about this. Marry anybody else. I married a welder."

(SillyFilly)

"Here's me with an eye-roll. Here's me with another. Thanks for your question. It's the best laugh I've had all day."

(PretzelGal)

"Where I am, most of the docs are married to other docs. I don't know any nurses married to MDs. Around here we tend to marry computer geeks and teachers."

(SmilinEyes)

"When I was a little girl that's exactly what I thought I would do. But now I can't imagine what it would be like, married to 90% of the docs I know. Stuck up and constantly bitchy, male or female. No thanks."

(ShandyLynn)

"My ex-wife married a male nurse and they seem pretty happy. I think he keeps her grounded to the real world."

(Kathy)

"I used to think about it. There was one resident in particular I really liked. Then I found him in the linen closet with a nurse-ho and that ended that."

(EricaBSN)

"Nuh, uh. Heck no. No. Not if doctors were the only males left on the planet. Hell no. Did I say no yet? No."

(Hallie)

"Just can't imagine a woman these days thinking an MD is a good catch. Some people must be stuck in a time warp. Maybe they haven't been around enough of them. Med school starts their mind-bend and health care finishes it off. Who needs an attitude-Andy with three ex-wives?"

(BoarderLVN)

"I'd marry a podiatrist if he'd play with my feet."

(WiseWomanRN)

"We're way too smart around here. I honestly don't know a single female who thinks a doctor would be a great long-term relationship."

(Sissy)

"Yes, I have two girlfriends who married doctors. They've both moved away to follow the men's careers. What I'd be curious to know is how many male nurses are with female doctors. That would be an interesting study."

(Lupa)

"No way. If I wanted to have anything to do with a doctor's life, I would have become one. Don't want to do it; don't want to be married to it."

(VivaRN)

"I work with a few women who seem hell-bent on getting together with physicians. At best they wind up 'getting it on' but nothing more. The docs just move on to the next starry-eyed twit. At our place it's the same group of doctors, constantly making the rounds. Some women have no class at all."

(Flo)

"Give me a break. I have two sisters, two aunts, a father and a grandmother, all of whom are nurses. Not one of them will have anything to do with a doctor. And I wouldn't touch one with nine-foot stick."

(Ironey)

"It's fun having a partner who's also into health care. 'My' doctor is far more people-oriented than the computer geek I was first married to. I admit mine is a rare find."

(KatLPN)

"My best friend chased that fairytale life. She married a cardiologist. The guy was so cheap he put her on an allowance. She

had to account for every dime. He eventually left her for a nurse. A few years later he left the nurse and married a secretary he was having an affair with. Now, do you want to hear about his kids and how screwed up they are?"
(JackieBSN)

"I'm almost afraid to admit that I married a doctor and we've been wonderfully happy for 16 years. I am proud to be his wife."
(SPeel)

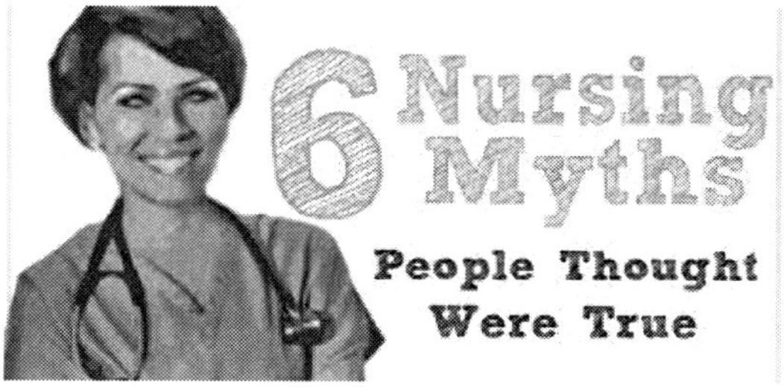

"In our large teaching hospital we like it when our women date these guys. Then they treat us better. We had one who thought he was too good to even return our calls to him when patients were dying. We were 'mere nurses.' His nurse girlfriend (now his wife) set him straight and made a fairly human doctor out of him. We buy her food."
(Charity)

"Well, most of the physicians I know are pleasant, but I cannot imagine a relationship with someone who is gone 18 hours a day."
(BooRN)

"My father is a doctor so maybe that's why I don't see the glamour in it at all. We have married neurologists who constantly hit on the women here. We have another MD with five kids and a wife going from one affair to the other. What, do *you* want to marry a doctor?"
(Sue)

"Never married one myself. I got their number very early in the game. Too egotistical and self-centered for me. I married a cute construction-type who has never let me down and puts our relationship first. There may be a doctor out there who prioritizes his family, but I haven't met one yet."
(MikesMom)

"My cousin is married to a urologist. He actually chose his specialty so he would have regular hours. They have the whole package. My best friend is married to an MD and although I love both of them and they seem happy, the more time goes on, the more I can see how he belittles her intelligence in front of people. I think that's just awful. She has dedicated her whole life to him."

(Leanne)

"My father is a terrific surgeon but a lousy dad. It took me years to realize what a cad he is, calling nurses 'honey' and touching them for fun. I work in the same hospital he does and I know he's been screwing around for years. Oh, well. I got lucky and married the sexiest plumber alive."

(Anklet)

"The 'nice' physician is still the exception and not the rule, in my experience."

(NancyNurse)

"I never had the slightest interest in marrying a doctor. The ones that showed interest in me were total jerks. My dreams came true with my husband of 20 years. He's a lumber broker!"

(Fiesty Nurse)

"Your question will spark anger in a lot of nurses, I'm sure. None of the qualities of these doctors are anything I'd want to marry into. My husband is a firefighter and he treats me as an equal."

(Fergus 51)

"You couldn't pay me enough money to marry any of the MDs I work with."

(Burger 914)

"The only doctors around here who treat nurses with respect are either gay or very old. Either way, marriage ain't an option."

(ErlinNP)

"I can honestly say that there were a handful of women in my class who really did plan on snagging a doc with money. Then they graduated and started working around them. Every single wannabe-wife did an about face."

(NurzwitFaith)

"Any fool who thinks they want to marry an MD hasn't met enough of these ingrates to hold a logical opinion."
(RitaPed)

"Yeah, right. In school the conversation often turned to dating a "nice, handsome doctor." Then we all found out that you won't meet one with both of those traits. On my floor of 22, five are married to firefighters; three to police officers and three to medics. We all met on the job. It seems we're just drawn to those rescue-types."
(JennieBSN)

"If that's your teenage fairytale it'll fade away eventually, like a bad case of pimples. I've heard too many of these guys yelling at their wives and girlfriends over the phone. No way would I live that way. It's bad enough to be treated like a second-class citizen by somebody else's ass of a husband."
(MistyMay)

"I didn't reply to your question initially because I couldn't stop my eyes from rolling around in my head long enough to type. Marry a doctor? Not on your life. I married a techno-weenie and I could not be happier. I honestly pity the bimbos who think they will ever be treated as well as they expect to be."
(BeaButter)

"Nothing looks more ridiculous in a hospital than a doe-eyed female coming down with white-coat fever. Where I work I've overheard MDs talking about 'working the nurse rotations,' i.e. 'have you done nurse Amber yet?'"
(Erin95)

"If you do decide to start dating one of these jackasses, please do yourself a favor and keep it to yourself. Otherwise, you'll soon find out you're just the most recent lady in a uniform to get used and dumped."
(MargoPostOp)

"Well, my best friend is a podiatry resident and he treats everybody really well. So they're not all self-possessed jerks. Just most of them."
(CashewLPN)

"I got a little offended when I saw your question. So many people think that's the real reason a woman wants to become a nurse. Plain stupid."

AnnieBSN)

"Can't speak for anyplace else, but here in South Florida it's nurse/ medic and nurse/cop. Some types just go together, like models and rock stars. I'm engaged to an MBA who works for FedEx. No medical background at all. Perfect!"

(ERDiva)

"I was married to a cop for 18 years. Marry a doctor? Not! Somebody's been reading too many Harlequin novels. I'd guess only one in ten doctors is even worth talking to. Condescending, rude and unapologetic males. The female docs aren't much fun either. They screw up and then yell at the nurse. And to think that in school I was taught to stand up when they enter the room and offer them my chair. That'll be the day."

(LessonLPN)

"I work in a small hospital and I know them all. I wouldn't get anywhere near even one of them. I treat them like the alien life-forms they are."

(JoolsDoc)

"Time for you to sit down and listen. If you marry a resident, you'll get dumped when they pass their boards. If you marry a divorced doc you'll help pay his alimony. In about five years he'll trade you in for the new hot thing in Post Op. Trust me. The only male more narcissistic than an MD is an airline pilot, and either way you're gonna' crash and burn. The women doctors can be impossible. Do yourself a favor and ask around."

(NormaRay)

"You're definitely going to get slammed for this question. Have you worked with these people? Have you spent any professional time with them at all? Most med students are pretty nice and they'll treat you like a peer. But docs will flirt with you in the lounge and then treat you like dirt out on the floor. I'm engaged to a sports bar manager. A doctor? Never happen."

(MaineChick)

"Not me nor anybody I hang out with. We've been around too many. Personally, I married a computer geek."
(PRN)

"I dunno. So many physicians seem to graduate from asshole U. My friend's husband is a family practitioner and he's a decent guy. But she's a captain in the Air Force so he might be afraid to mess with her. She could pick up the phone and have a missile torch him driving down the highway."
(BabyRN)

"Plumbers are better men, period. And Lord knows they wash their hands more often."
(RadBSN)

"I work with a wonderful group of doctors. Really terrific guys. But there is no way I'd get involved with any of them."
(SRC)

"Well, well, well. So you think nurses want to marry these people? The only nurse I ever met who was happily married was a male med/surg with a lady OB/GYN. That's one in 35 years. So you tell me. Do yourself a favor: choose a partner, not a control freak."
(TeenaTrainer)

"Hey, kids. Take it from one who did – marry an MD, that is. Physicians spend 10 years learning how to always be right. The overwhelming number of people working around them are females who have been taught to never argue, ever. If you think that a male doc going home to his wife at night will suddenly flip that "because I say so" switch off, you're living in Michael Jackson's Neverland. Oh, I forgot. His doctor killed him."
(LynnRN)

"A good friend of mine is married to a cardiologist and it seems to work well for them. I personally had my chance and then Providence intervened. Thank God we broke up when we did. He is now known as the jackass of the clinic."
(Cyndy)

"I my case, I wasn't a woman looking for a doctor. I just happened to meet the love of my life in a grocery store and it turned

out he was a med student. I love him for who he is, not what he's going to be."
(AllHeartRN)

"Well, these days half the people in med school are women, so the tables they are a turning. The question is, will male nurses be interested in lady docs? Stay tuned."
(CarritTop)

"I'm pretty sure my girlfriend would get mad if I married a doctor, so I guess I won't."
(PillBill)

"The best doctor on our floor is a woman, and she's now engaged to one of the security guards. I know this has nothing to do with your question, but I thought it shows how love really works. Job titles aren't the final word."
(Larry)

"In our hospital they're either old and crotchety or Indian and strange around females. It's enough to turn a girl celibate."
(Lunacy)

"The most attractive males around here are the techs."
(FireEyes)

"Marry a doctor? Yikes! What a strange thought."
(Agnes in Admin)

"Become a nurse to marry a doctor. Hmmm. I'd put that in the category of little girls wearing adult clothes."
(Sunshine)

"Lord, this is hilarious. The only people that want to marry an ego-on-wheels are the nuts who don't know enough nurses for intelligent feedback."
(MarvelousMarva)

"The only doc I'll ever love is my son. Yes, he's an intern."
(Abby)

"I have two nurse friends who were married to physicians. They were both replaced by newer versions last year. Like cell phones. Tell you anything at all?"
(ChiTownMSN)

"Becoming a nurse to marry a doctor? Isn't that like joining the Army to go to Afghanistan to marry an officer? Who in hell thinks like that?"
(PillMoma)

"Sorry but no. I snagged myself a really cool mechanic. Great guy and free car repairs for life."
(NurseBluBear)

"Can't stand them at work. Why would I want one at home?"
(Valerie)

"Well, there was this pediatric pulmonologist. Jeez. I'd marry him just to hear that voice of his. Yum."
(AR RN)

"The first thing my grandmother said to me when she heard I was in nursing school was, 'Oh, good. Now you can meet a nice doctor.' Uh, no."
(Shenanigans)

"My aunt is a psych nurse and she married a psychiatrist. They've been together for 30 years and are crazy about each other. Okay, so maybe 'crazy' is the operative word. So we know it can work."
(LizzTech)

"My second husband is a doctor. I always refused to date the ones I worked around, but damn. I fell for my best friend."
(Proud2BNursing)

"After some thought I decided to comment on this subject. My wife is an MD and I am a homemaker/RN. My wife comes home exhausted and testy and often depressed. Work takes everything she has and I get whatever is left of her energy and attention. If I try to discuss our problems it always leads to a fight. The last time we had sex was six months ago. We have a decent marriage in most regards, but I have to say the medical profession sucks the life out of people."
(Ariko)

"I've been married to a man who is an MD for 32 years now. Best I can say is that we have a good marriage. I never was going to marry any doctor – I saw too much of how they change after residency. I got lucky and got a good one. I think it helps that he's a pediatrician."

(Eileen)

"Oh, hell no! But I'd marry a veterinarian. They know all about how to handle lovable little creatures."

(Leslie)

"I narrowly escaped marrying a plastic surgeon. Thank God I didn't. Wow, did he turn out to be a putz on wheels."

(NurseDi)

"In my experience, 99% of physicians cheat on their wives. Sad but true. So I'd never think of getting involved with one because they just can't be trusted."

(Yadi)

"I only know one physician who treats women the way they should be treated. Of course, he's a transsexual, so even though his patients don't know it, he used to be one."

(Marla MSN)

"My husband says he's the Doctor of Love. Does that count?"

(Kornflake)

Well, we think that just about covers it.

Immutable Law #3
Becoming a nurse to marry a doctor?
Unadulterated fiction.

"Maybe we'll get lucky. Maybe God'll come down and pull us all over for speeding."

—Pervis Lee

Chapter Four

Lights & sirens, bells & whistles

The fantasy can start early in life. We thank reporter Rico R. Reed in South Carolina for the following submission:

Student wins EMS essay contest; gets a fast ambulance ride

Imagine being in the second grade and one day you are picked up by an ambulance instead of a school bus. The next thing you know, you're pulling up on the playground with lights & sirens going, as your teachers and classmates stand cheering you on. Sound like a dream? Actually it was a dream that came true for three lucky Charleston County second-graders.

The students were winners of the County EMS coloring contest. The theme for this year's contest was, *"What Does EMS Mean to Me?"*

Dalia Dalili of Whiteside Elementary won first place and got a ride in the ambulance on May 23. Her class also got a visit from 'Andy the Ambulance Man' who answered everybody's questions about EMS. But the best part was when Dalia got to ride in the patient compartment with a real paramedic. She had the opportunity to handle some specialized equipment and even talked with a 911 dispatcher. And the very best part of all was that she got to turn on the red lights & siren as they pulled up to the school.

Program spokesman Archie Hirschmann said he welcomed the chance to coordinate the event with the children. The annual program is sponsored by the Crayon Team of Charleston County, a volunteer group of EMS personnel dedicated to public recognition of emergency services.

"As much as these kids loved that siren," Hirschmann said, "I expect we're creating a whole generation of future EMT recruits."

❖

"We suffer from 'Maximal Response' disease and red lights and sirens are the symptoms."
Jeff J. Clawson MD.

❖

So maybe now we can stop wondering why the profession is chock-full of Rescue Randys who can't keep their grubby hands off the siren switch. It is time to be fair and balanced about another reality. What follows is 1% of EMS tragedies over the last two years alone. Sadly, they represent 1100 others that can be found if you research any other year, in *Accident Archives*:

Retired Fire Chief dies after colliding with high-speed ambulance

In the city of Stanford Kentucky a deadly collision has taken the life of a former fire chief of Lincoln County.

Deputy Coroner Tony Floro reported that Mr. Walter Manuel, age 79 of Stanford, was pronounced dead at the scene of a two-vehicle crash, at the intersection of U.S. 27 and Lancaster Street. Police Chief Keith Middleton told reporters that the collision was the result of a Stanford EMS unit transporting a patient Code-3 and proceeding through a red light. Middleton stated that although the ambulance had its red lights and siren activated at the time, it did not stop or slow sufficiently to avoid cross traffic.

All three members of the EMS team, as well as the patient, were injured but are expected to survive.

❖

Heart patient in Houston ambulance killed in crash

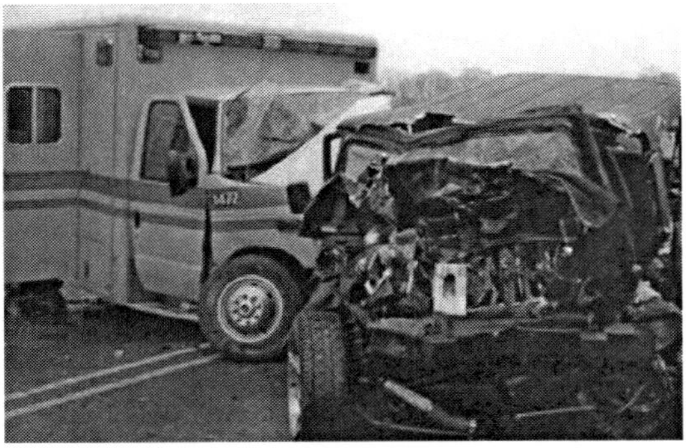

This happens 3-5 times a day, every day of the year (Photo credit: Lance Teeson)

A man died Monday morning after a pickup struck the ambulance that was taking him to the hospital, authorities said. The Ford F-150 collided with a *Houston Fire Department* ambulance about 9:20 a.m. in the 9800 block of Bissonnet, according to Houston police. Police say the ambulance was traveling with its revolving lights and siren at the time the collision occurred.

❖

Six injured in Georgia ambulance crash

The driver of a pickup truck which collided with an ambulance in Dougherty County remains in the hospital tonight. The incident happened in the 1800 block of County Line Road.

Police say Christopher Barfield was driving a pick-up truck Saturday when he turned left, in front of a Dougherty County EMS unit that was passing another truck.

Authorities say EMT Erskin Livingston, who was driving the ambulance, as well as his passenger, Victor Allen, suffered unknown injuries. An adult passenger in the truck was also treated for minor injuries. Police say a two- month-old and a one-year-old child also in the truck were slightly injured.

"When you see an emergency vehicle approaching you from the rear the best thing you can do is to go to the right, allow us to pass. It makes it a lot easier on everybody," said Corporal Ted Wertz with the Dougherty County Police Department.

The ambulance was responding to a traffic collision and had lights and siren on at the time.

❖

Four injured after ambulance overturns in New York

Four people were injured on a Thursday evening in August when a high-speed ambulance overturned after colliding with a car at an intersection. Early reports indicate the ambulance, which had two medics and a patient inside at the time, crashed at about 5:45 p.m. and flipped on its side at the intersection of 3rd Ave and 61st Street in Brooklyn. The driver of the car was also hurt and all four were taken to a local hospital. Their conditions are not as yet known.

❖

Father and son seriously hurt in crash with a fire truck

At 9:05 a.m. Thursday a call rang out for a man suffering chest pains, so four firefighters jumped into their truck and sped out of Station 41 near Ridgeway Highway in Memphis, Tennessee.

Barely seven minutes later, at the intersection of Ridgeway and Interstate 240, the fire truck collided with a white Ford Taurus, critically injuring a 29-year-old mother and her one-year-old son.

The child was ejected from the car, police said, while the woman was trapped inside. Further details are unavailable at this time.

❖

Two EMTs, one patient killed in South Georgia ambulance wreck

Both members of an EMS team as well as their patient, were killed early Thursday when the ambulance in which they were riding collided with a jackknifing tractor-trailer on a South Georgia highway, authorities said.

The crash happened about 5:00 a.m. on route 32 in Irwin County.

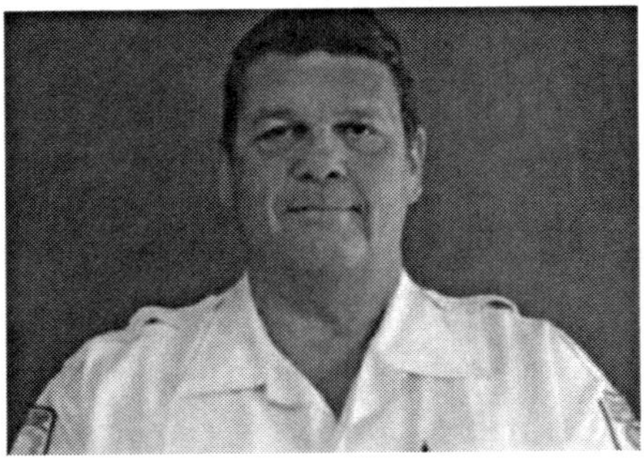

Randall Whiddon, EMS Chief (Photo by son Ben Whiddon)

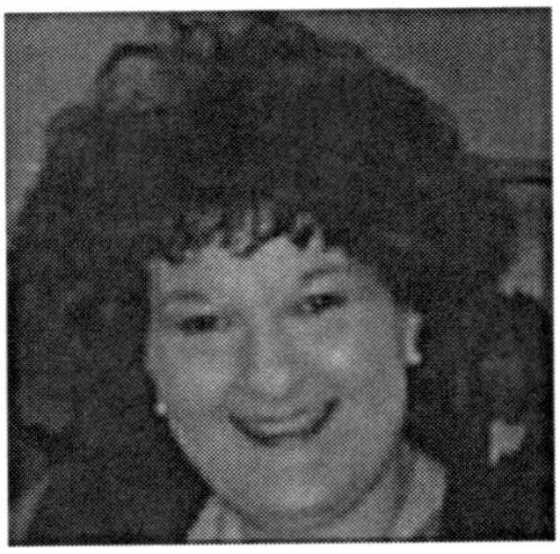

EMT Teresa Davis Gurley (Photo by her family)

Georgia State Patrol spokeswoman Franka Young said the tractor-trailer and a passenger car were apparently headed westbound on the two-lane road when the eastbound ambulance from Coffee County approached with lights and siren activated.

The car pulled off the roadway in front of the large truck, to yield to the approaching ambulance," Young said. "The tractor-trailer jackknifed across the center line to avoid hitting the car, but went into the path of the ambulance."

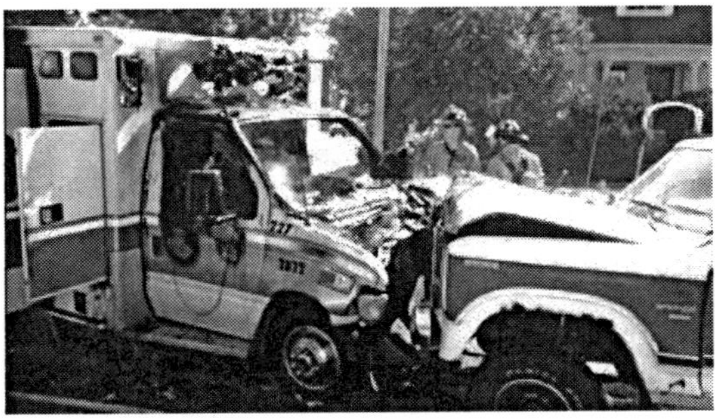

50 times a year – on average – we run into each other

She identified the medic-driver of the ambulance as Teresa Davis Gurley, age 44, of Axson. The medic tending the patient was Randall Whiddon, 56, of Ashburn. The patient was identified as Charles Smith, age 65, of Tifton.

❖

One dead, five injured after crash involving ambulance

A 63-year-old North Las Vegas resident is dead and five other people are injured after a crash involving an ambulance on Tuesday morning.

The crash happened at about 10:30 a.m. at the intersection of Decatur Road and Craig Road in northeast Las Vegas.

Police say witnesses indicated the ambulance was driving through the intersection with lights and sirens active when a Nissan Frontier entered the intersection on a green light, striking the ambulance.

The ambulance, which was taking a woman to the hospital, rolled over on its left side.

That woman later died at *Mountain View Hospital*. It is not yet known whether she died as a result of the crash or pre-existing medical conditions. A North Las Vegas firefighter, an EMT and two *MedicWest* personnel who were in the ambulance at the time of the crash, were all taken to *University Medical Center* with unknown injuries.

❖

Driver of ambulance cited in crash that killed U-W doctor

The driver of the *Meriter Hospital* ambulance that crashed in July, killing a doctor onboard, was fined for failure to keep the vehicle under control, according to the final incident report released last week.

According to the report the ambulance, equipped for newborn patients, was going to Appleton to pick up a baby for specialized surgery when it crashed about 12:35 p.m. on July 10. No criminal charges will be filed, said Captain Rick Olig of the *Fond du Lac Sheriff's Office.*

Ross Fleming, age 62, a retired Madison Police Officer, is believed to inadvertently have driven into a culvert at a high rate of speed and flipped the vehicle over on its side.

Killed was Doctor Stanley Phillips III, 32. Doctor Phillips had recently finished medical school training. Two other medical staff in the back of the ambulance were treated and released. Another remained at *UW Hospital* for several days after surgery.

❖

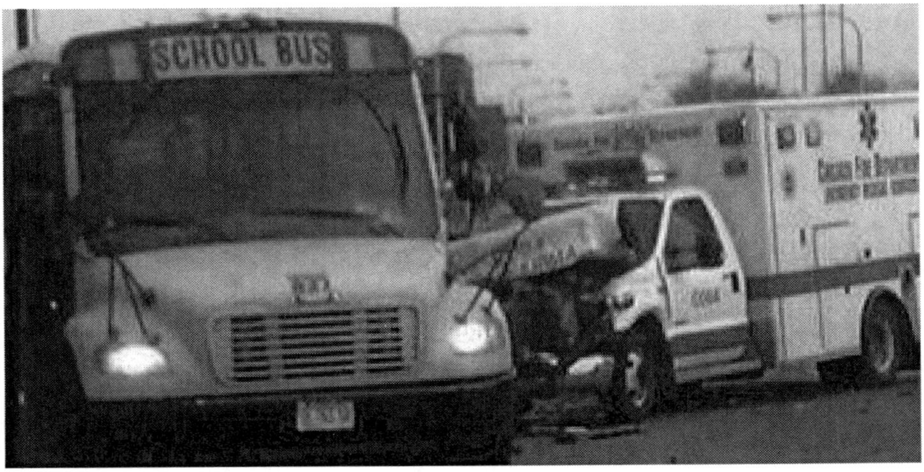

This one hit a school bus
(Photo credit: Lee Whitmore)

Five injured in ambulance crash in Davie, Florida

Five people suffered minor injuries in a crash involving an ambulance and two other vehicles in September, Davie city police said.

The collision happened around 6 p.m. at Oakes Road and South State Road 7. An *American Medical Response* ambulance was transporting a patient when it collided with a van and a small car, then flipped onto its passenger side, according to the initial report.

Traffic on southbound State Road 7 was detoured around the crash scene for over an hour. The injured were treated at the scene and all but one were taken to *Broward Health Medical Center*.

❖

Pittsburgh ambulance collides with motorcycle; three people injured

Two emergency medical technicians were injured on a Friday night in October after their ambulance collided with a motorcyclist along a local Pennsylvania highway.

Early reports by police on scene indicate the motorcyclist suffered serious injuries and was taken to a local hospital in critical condition.

One of the injured EMTs was pregnant, according to the report. Her condition is not known at this time.

❖

Four people hurt in New Jersey ambulance crash

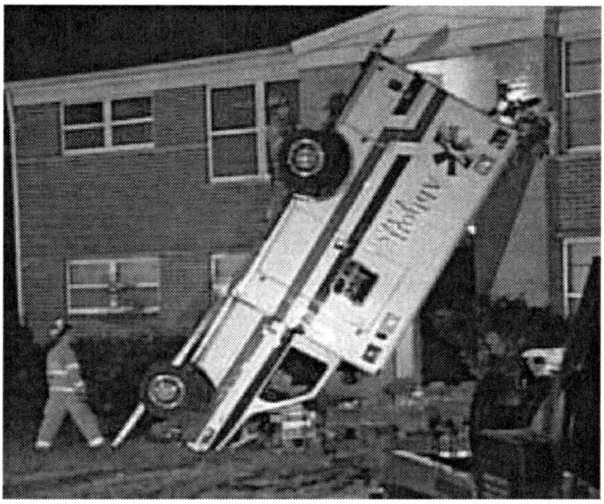

Just when you think you've seen it all (Photo: Kirkwood Missouri Fire Dept.)

A total of four people were reported injured in an accident involving a Camden County ambulance in May.

According to Gloucester Township Police, a resident's car was exiting a private driveway when it backed into the street in front of a *Gloucester Township EMS* unit, causing the ambulance to hit the vehicle at "moderate speed." The ambulance was transporting a patient to a local hospital at the time of the crash. All three EMTs, as well as the driver of the car, were taken to local hospitals with various injuries. The condition of the patient being transported is not known.

❖

Two killed in Cass County ambulance collision

Two people are dead and two others critically injured after a crash involving an ambulance in Cass County, about 20 miles east of Lincoln Nebraska, late on a Tuesday night in June.

Authorities said a 2002 Ford Ranger was traveling east on Highway 34 when it crossed the center line and collided head-on with a *Weeping Water Rescue* ambulance. The ambulance was on its way to a hospital in Lincoln with a patient with lights and sirens activated.

The Jaws of Life was needed to extricate the driver of the ambulance, identified as Bob Hanes, 51. Mr. Hanes died shortly after arriving at *Bryan Medical Center*. The driver of the Ford Ranger, 24-year-old William J. Whitlatch from rural Syracuse, was pronounced dead at the scene.

Two EMTs, including Hanes' 30-year-old daughter, Melissa, and 46-year-old James "Beau" Flint, suffered critical injuries in the crash.

❖

San Francisco ambulance crash injures three

A female Paramedic and two other people were injured when an SUV collided with an ambulance one morning in January. The incident happened in San Francisco's Laurel Heights neighborhood about 7:55 in the morning, according to a fire department spokeswoman.

The crash happened at Geary Boulevard and Spruce Street. The ambulance was en route to a medical call and was traveling east on Geary Boulevard with its siren on at the time. It was struck by a vehicle traveling north on Spruce Street, fire spokeswoman Mindy Talmadge said.

The Paramedic, who was seated on the passenger side of the ambulance, was taken to a hospital to be evaluated.

Two people in the other vehicle were also hospitalized, Talmadge said. She did not know the extent of the victims' injuries.

❖

Fatal ambulance crash results in lawsuit

The family of a 75-year-old woman killed in a 2009 vehicle collision involving an ambulance in July is seeking damages from the *Sellersburg Volunteer Fire Department* in an ongoing civil trial in Clark County.

Opal Couch of Jeffersonville was killed after a SVFD ambulance of *Clark County Indiana EMS*, struck the side of her Lincoln passenger car about on July 4 in an intersection on Lewis and Clark Parkway.

The driver of the ambulance, Travis Herthel, testified in court that Couch's vehicle was fully stopped at the intersection when he proceeded through the red light. The victim was struck when she apparently started a left turn in front of the ambulance.

Herthel reported that he was traveling at "emergency pace" with the ambulance siren and lights activated.

Herthel said on the day of the accident the roads were wet after hours of light rain and the road condition resulted in a more severe impact.

❖

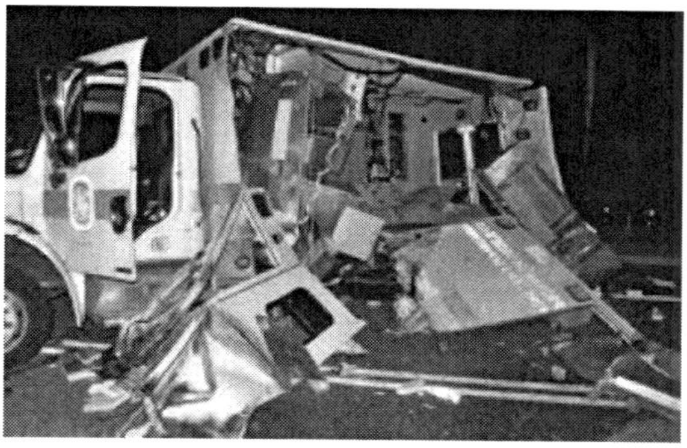

Does Code-3 save lives? Think twice before you answer (Photo: Prince George's County Sheriff, Maryland)

Jury to decide if Utah EMT was negligent

Sean Reed Applonie is charged with negligent homicide in the death more than a year ago of a motorist who was struck by his North Davis Fire District ambulance near Ogden one year ago. Applonie, 28, has pleaded not guilty to the misdemeanor charge. After hitting the Buick, police said, his ambulance then struck two other cars.

Arline H. Logan, 88, was killed in the collision July 6, just east of *Ogden Regional Medical Center*. In all, six people were injured, including two of Applonie's fellow EMTs and his passenger.

Although numerous questions remain, officials agree there is no question the westbound ambulance was operating with red lights and siren at the time.

❖

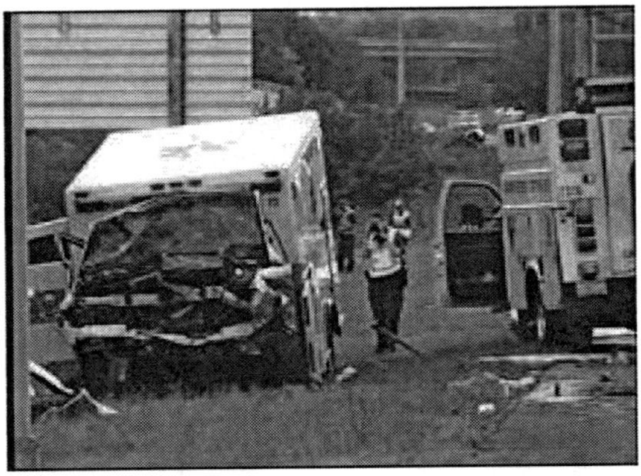

This one killed a medic and his elderly patient (Photo: WKRN TV Nashville)

Mississippi fire chief killed in wreck with deputy sheriff

A Newton County volunteer fire chief was killed on a Saturday night in July in a crash while responding to another collision.

Greenfield's Chief Mickey Yates' pickup truck collided with a deputy sheriff's vehicle. The pickup overturned and Chief Yates was ejected. The Mississippi Highway Patrol said the deputy sheriff did not suffer life-threatening injuries. The cause of the crash is under investigation.

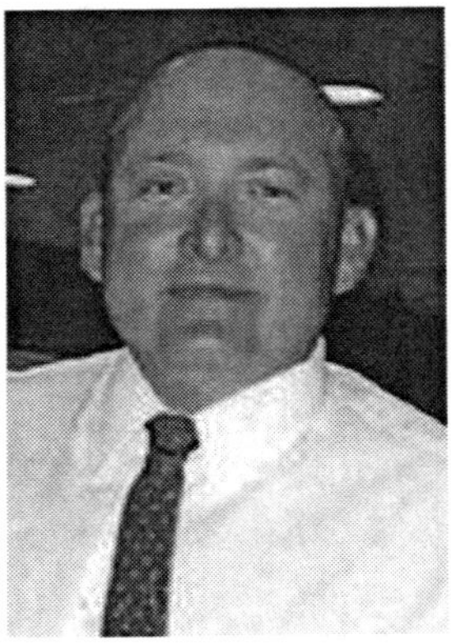

Greenfield MS. Chief Yates (Photo Credit: Sanctuary of Mary)

❖

Los Angeles Fire Chief loses job after EMS response-times scandal

Los Angeles Mayor Eric Garcetti announced the decision in October to replace the city's fire chief after a tumultuous 18 months administering the city's largest emergency rescue agency.

Chief Brian Cummings, who announced his retirement immediately afterwards, apparently never recovered from a systems audit last March. That audit reported that the fire department's 911 response time data was not an accurate accounting of the facts. The data made it appear that ambulances were arriving faster to rescues than they actually did.

A *Los Angeles Times* investigation had previously documented widespread delays in EMS dispatching; routine failures to summon the closest EMS teams from surrounding areas when needed, as well as serious disparities in getting rescuers to life-threatening emergencies in different parts of the city. According to Garcetti, none of these flaws in the system were appropriately addressed in Chief Cummings' routine correspondence with the City Council.

❖

Two Florida paramedics injured in rescue truck crash

Two Paramedics had to be extricated through the front windshield of their rescue truck after they were struck broadside by a car near Tampa last October.

Police say Terry McFarland, age 47, the driver of the other vehicle, was traveling westbound on First Avenue when he ran a red light at 2:20 a.m., striking the rescue vehicle. Both Paramedics as well as a passenger in McFarland's car suffered minor injuries. McFarland, who was uninjured, was arrested for driving under the influence and driving on a suspended license.

❖

Texas ambulance crash injures two EMTs

A high-speed crash between a *Denison Fire Department* ambulance and a car left two EMTs and the driver of the car injured in November. The ambulance was responding to an emergency call when the collision occurred, according to a Denison police spokesman.

All three people involved were taken to a nearby hospital for treatment, and in accordance with departmental policy, both EMTs underwent mandatory drug and alcohol tests.

❖

Pickup truck broadsided by ambulance in Santa Maria

A collision involving a *Santa Barbara County EMS* unit resulted in three injuries, according to Santa Maria police officials.

The report states that an *American Medical Response* ambulance was en route to an emergency medical call when it struck the driver's side of a Chevy truck at about 4:00 p.m. on April 3. The seriousness of the injuries of the EMTs and the driver of the truck has not yet been reported.

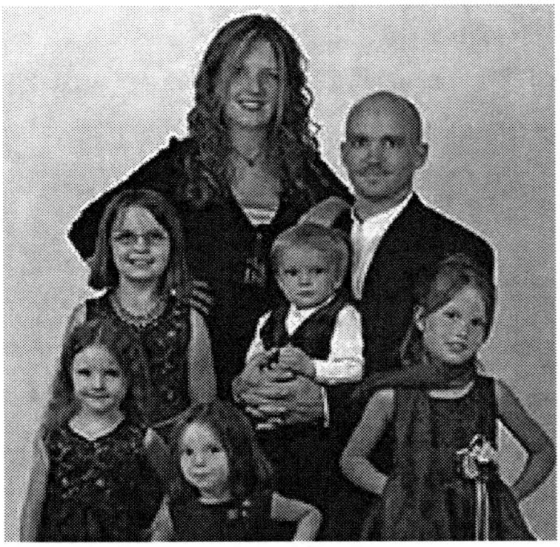

EMT Tammy Mundell,
wife and mom
(Photo credit: Maverick)

❖

Phoenix Arizona EMT killed in ambulance collision

An emergency medical technician for *Southwest Ambulance* died at the scene of a crash near Casa Grande, south of Phoenix.

According to Arizona Highway Patrol, 29-year-old Tammy Mundell and her partner, Sandra Williams, were transporting an inmate from the Arizona State Prison when it collided at the intersection of state highways 87 and 287.

Williams, who was tending to the patient in the back of the ambulance at the time of the crash, was airlifted to *Maricopa Medical Center* in critical condition. A state corrections officer and the inmate were also taken to regional hospitals.

Mrs. Mundell, who was eight months pregnant at the time of her death, leaves a husband and five children.

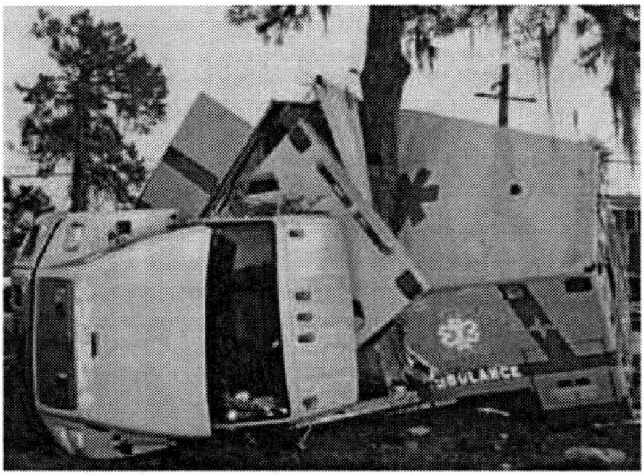

How much proof do you suppose you need?
(Photo credit: NIOSH Safety Investigators, Florida)

❖

Because you chose us for your dose of reality therapy, we will inform you right now that Code-3 (lights & siren) ambulance responses happen thousands of times a day for no good reason. In spite of what plenty of fine folks have come to believe – maybe even you – the fact is EMS 'shock & awe' is rarely a significant influencer in saving lives by getting to the patient faster. Neither does it usually improve patient outcomes by getting them to the ER a blink or two quicker. More than a few studies have shown that – contrary to the convictions of the EMS world – Code-3 driving puts medics; their patients; other responders and the public in unnecessary peril. So much so that, by all measurable criteria, the routine practice quite possibly generates as much trauma and death as it prevents. Now, how smart can that be, really?

The tradition of flipping on lights & sirens by ambulance teams has, over seven decades, morphed into a reflex so axiomatic that few people on either side of the EMS equation give it much real thought. It just is. Code-3 has been elevated to a sacramental practice which now sports all the hallmarks of – as comedian Stephen Colbert likes to say – 'truthiness.' It must be right because it feels right. Code-3 is religious dogma because, well, by God, it's an emergency. It appeals to our sense of righteousness. "Let's go! Fast is good, faster is better!"

No, actually, it isn't.

One needs to look no further for proof of this breathless, need-for-speed zealotry than the bizarre creation of the 'Golden Hour.' This medical myth was the brainchild of Doctor R. Adams Cowley, who founded the *Shock Trauma Center* in Baltimore Maryland. The man was an exceptional physician; a visionary; a pioneer in trauma care and a key player in integrating medical helicopters into EMS. Yet his Golden Hour pronouncement – however well-intentioned it partially was – has been proven nearly worthless as a functional aspect of patient delivery. But not, unfortunately, before it was swallowed up by so many for so long that it was patently embarrassing to those of us who viscerally knew better. Here's Tim Noonan, whose educational EMS blog is called, *The Rogue Medic*:

"The 'Golden Hour' is just another example of problems we have with protocols. It substitutes an artificial deadline (60 minutes) in place of Paramedic judgment in an individual situation. The Golden Hour is another example of the medical profession not believing Paramedics are capable of critical thinking and good judgment."

So true.

Doctor Adams Cowley, the man responsible for some of the finest aspects of trauma care in the 1960s, was also at the helm of one of the greatest scams in emergency delivery. The crux of his theory was, well, let's use his words:

"There is a golden hour between life and death," he preached. "If you are critically injured you have less than 60 minutes to survive. You might not die right then; it may be three days or two weeks later. But something has happened in your body in that 60 minutes that is irreparable."

The brightest emergency physicians we know shake their heads sadly at such self-serving pablum. But of course they never speak up.

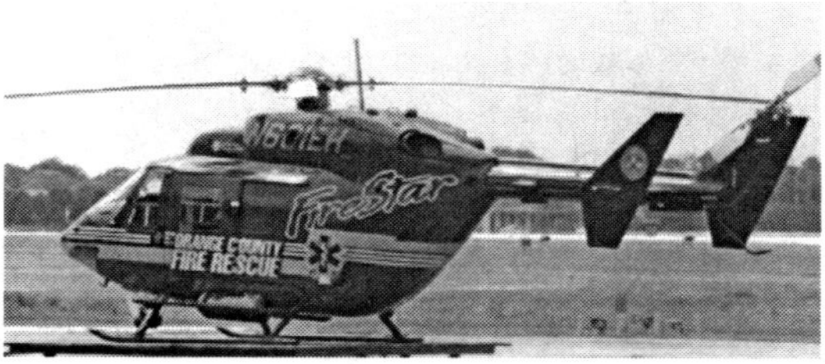

Orange County Florida's nifty air ambulance
(We thank Ken Marx for the photo)

We never had the pleasure of meeting Adams Cowley at any of the EMS conferences we attended. But if we had, we would have told him we absolutely love his helicopters. Then we would asked him if he truly believed such nonsense, or if he hadn't just created his Golden Hour to convince a medically ignorant citizenry; a gullible congress and a chomping-at-the-bit EMS choir, that the state of Maryland needed millions to fund its helicopters and that he was the one to lead the air cavalry.

The indiscriminate application of the Golden Hour helped prime the frenzy that when it comes to first aid – speed is the need. This simply is not true. Allow me to paraphrase how educated, clearer minds weigh in:

The type of medical problem; the age and underlying health of the victim; the mysterious *vigor* with which some victims can bounce back, are all huge components in what is known as the patient's *physiologic reserve.* This nearly unquantifiable asset can be strained and drained by any number of other factors, before, during and after the incident that generates the 911 call. Human ability to recover is a broad-spectrum commodity, and it varies from one person to the next. People are not born wearing a physiologic reserve meter on their foreheads. There is absolutely no logical reason for caregivers to believe that rushing every accident victim to a trauma center will improve their outcomes – if only they meet the magic, 60-minute Heaven's Gate time clock. Because by now we have all heard the stories of one man surviving a nail gun shot to the brain, while another poor chap dies after stepping on a toothpick in the carpet.

Physiologic reserve.

An excellent report on just this subject was issued last year by the *Arizona Department of Health & Services.* Their research determined there is "considerable overuse of air ambulances for trauma victims."

The Golden Hour is one man's fantasy and has no place whatsoever in an EMS delivery system. Yet thousands of my otherwise bright colleagues continue to bow to its goofy gospel.

But Lord knows "rushed to the hospital" makes the news and wow! EMS helicopters – the most lethal form of transportation on earth. Are they sexy, or what?

❖

Just because something feels like warm and fuzzy common sense, doesn't mean that it is. In five out of eight lights & siren responses you happen to witness on city streets on a given day, those fine folks in uniform are dashing off to no true emergency at all. In nearly every one of the other three cases, arriving one, two or three minutes later would have no downside whatsoever.

As far back as 20 years ago, research conducted for the *Annals of Emergency Medicine* determined that patient transportation time from the scene of an incident to the emergency room, in a given city, was 43 seconds slower without lights and sirens. And while this difference in ambulance time may seem important to the citizenry – it is certainly not important medically. In layman's terms, a vehicle delivering you to the ER 43 seconds faster, does not mean hospital staff can work magic within those extra seconds to improve your situation. In fact, five-to-ten minute delays are almost never clinically important either.

A few minutes saved were probably once clinically valuable in a fraction of cases, in the era when speed was all an ambulance had to offer. For the most part, detailed physical assessment and advanced-level intervention just did not happen with unskilled care providers of the times. But today there exists practically no circumstance where "a minute lost is a patient lost." In fact and in most cases, the first half-dozen things that a doctor and nurse would do, have already been done. That is what basic and advanced life support gets you. It's why we master medicine instead of drag racing.

For nigh on 40 years the eight-minute response time has been the platinum standard for the value of EMS to its community. The "we're quicker than the other guys" mentality has dominated practically every EMS contract conversation since *Emergency.* In the era of the Gold Rush the mantra of the macho was, "who's the fastest gun in the West?" In the outré world of EMS, it still is. Playing the speedy-medic card is – to a great extent – exactly how the largest EMS provider in the U.S. won all those lucrative contracts. *American Medical Response* succeeded in leveraging the fuzzy math of quicker ambulances, to convince 2,000+ communities that parking Paramedics on street corners means faster times and by default, a better way to do things.

Not even close. Quite the opposite, in fact. The unintended consequences are astronomical.

What it guarantees instead is a never-ending stream of twenty-something burned-out medics with often not much in the life-experience bucket, using the revolving door of *AMR* to gain a modicum of street cred while they shop for a 'real' job. And real positions – if you ask them – mean you're not parked at Poco Taco assuaging your stress with a burrito after treating a bloody mess. To the contrary, rescuers should be afforded the simple decency of being allowed to return to a crew quarters; take a shower and decompress from the god-awful mess they just experienced. Mind you, medics don't require much in order to do the job properly. A shower and a bunk, a fresh shirt and a padded cell would cut staff turn-over by 90%.

In the bizarre world of EMS, this nation's largest care provider subscribes to the same theory of staff hiring and turnover as McDonald's hamburgers: mediocrity works just fine, and we can always find new medics for less money when the experienced ones can't take it anymore.

And politicians – always in search of a quick fix for less money – buy this goofy pass at logic, hook, line and plumb bob. And ambulance providers – who need EMS contracts to survive – pretend speed is the need, and medics with two years experience are good enough. Wiser minds in this business know better. But even they tacitly approve private sector medics parked on street corners, trying very hard to catch a nap without catching a cootie. And trust me: you can have some truly spooky nightmares while lying on a ghost-ridden gurney in a parking lot.

Our antiquated, arranged marriage of 'quick response' to 'the best interest of the public' is but one aspect of health care that turns logic on its dizzy head. Distilled to its lowest common denominator, private carrier EMS has convinced you of this little mind-bend:

"Don't worry. We'll save you, even if it ends careers; trashes a noble profession; bankrupts half of us and kills people."

Indeed, the elevation of lights & sirens to sainthood is scribed for all to see in the highly respected *National Fire Protection Association* code book. Specifically, the *NFPA* states that early response units should take no longer than four minutes to get to any incident, on a quarterly average of 90% of the dispatches. Paramedics are mandated to be on scene within eight minutes. The basis of this thinking is that when a heart, brain or blood vessel goes into crisis mode, intervention within those narrow time frames is paramount. Yes, no one would argue that on those highly rare calls, a quicker response beats a slower response. We have no qualms with that. But just for balance, wrap your mind around this:

In the first week of February, 2011, Dallas was hosting Super Bowl XLV, where the Green Bay Packers would play the Pittsburgh Steelers. Three days before the game a monster storm clobbered the area with half a foot of snow and ice. The temperatures plunged and the storm was so extreme that *MedStar*, the area's largest EMS provider, made the unprecedented decision to suspend all Code-3 responses. In order to keep its fleet of 35 ambulances on the road and out of the ditch, every call was handled very, very slowly. Now, *MedStar* covers a 500 square mile service area of Texas with just under 1,000,000 residents. They can run 3,000 calls per week. During the storm period their dispatchers took in more than 1,700 calls: car crashes, chest pain, difficulty breathing, childbirth, frozen people, et al. One of their emergency calls was to Cowboy Stadium in Arlington, where several tons of ice slid off the roof and seriously injured seven people, with one critical. Still, no lights and sirens for two full days and two full nights.

In the weeks following the Super Bowl, *MedStar* operations staff had the time and the wisdom to compare their 911 results during the storm – with no lights and sirens – to normal 48-hour periods when they certainly were used. And they were as startled as anybody to discover that there was no measurable difference in patient outcomes.

This fact is worth repeating. *No lights and sirens on 700+ EMS calls during extraordinary weather. No measurable difference in patient outcomes.*

For some of us logic is nothing, if not a royal pain in the backside.

Now consider the flip side. The trauma and fatalities, the lawsuits, vehicle downtime, psychological harm to programs and families, is stunning. And the crashes occur with an almost preposterous frequency. Here is a peek at a 20-year study of what indiscriminate Code-3 driving buys us:

2-Decade Overview - EMS Crashes/Deaths/Injuries

Year	EMS Crashes	Deaths	Serious Injuries
1990	1002	12	506
1991	1275	18	337
1992	2865	25	752
1993	3350	16	1514
1994	1265	23	548
1995	3135	18	688
1996	1952	15	518
1997	2351	17	347
1998	2343	16	1750
1999	2288	9	902
2000	3160	15	1215
2001	2800	15	931
2002	2600	10	1402
2003	2268	16	1222
2004	1813	19	1186
2005	1452	24	1151
2006	2050	10	816
2007	2083	18	440
2008	2975	14	873
2009	1382	16	510
20 yrs	**44,409**	**326**	**17,608**

Some pretty grim math, don't you think?

Over the identical timeframe EMS vehicles experienced a higher frequency of crashes than fire apparatus and police units combined. This is a striking phenomenon when one considers that patrol cars travel five times as many miles per day as ambulances. Now consider this:

"EMS personnel have an occupational fatality rate of 9.6 per 100,000 workers per year, in transportation-related incidents. The death rate is 6.3 for police; 4.5 for firefighters and 2 for average citizens."

National Institute for Occupational Safety & Health

❖

It is time for my stubborn brethren to face reality. A few saved seconds here or there are literally inconsequential, compared to the trauma epidemic documented above. And an ambulance running "hot" as they say, is twice as likely to be involved in a fatal collision as one running at normal traffic speeds. One reason for this is that the siren itself is a highly limited warning device. Modern-day drivers with windows up and music on simply cannot hear a siren quickly enough to respond. From the EMS driver standpoint, well, we've been there more than 10,000 times. We can promise you that "running hot" is exciting. Because of this, it can mess with your head. And after you have done it a few hundred times, you are no longer even aware just how much you rationalize the risk.

From a patient care standpoint the siren has an unnecessarily negative impact on victims being transported, who are already as frightened as they have ever been in their lives. Physiologically, a fast ride in an ambulance can and often does cause spikes in heart rate, blood pressure and respirations, as well as irregular heartbeats on the EKG, none of which is a great idea.

So it is not hard to see what the overuse of lights & sirens does. We can also see what it does not do. No known study has demonstrated or even adequately suggested that Code-3 driving by ambulances saves lives. So what do we do instead?

You start by changing the paradigm:

- Begin teaching students from first grade exactly how to describe a 911 emergency in detail on the telephone
- Continue this training all the way through high school
- Add "911-speak" to the Driver Training curriculum
- Employ Paramedics and ER nurses as 911 dispatchers
- Use social media for massive public re-education programs. In at least 30% of the cases callers don't need an ambulance – they need a taxi. In another percentage of cases, they don't need an ER – they need an urgent care facility
- Educate, educate. Far too often, the problem is not found in EMS response times. It is, rather, in delayed calls in the first place
- Place automatic defibrillators in every public place, including on buses and in police cars
- Demonstrate the wisdom of not calling 911 as better options become implemented
- Ensure that the EMS driver makes the final speed deci-

sion. Not a dispatcher 10 miles away, and certainly not 'policy.'

❖

The cost to operate a fire truck can average $2,000 every time it leaves the station. A busy city apparatus can respond 12 times per day. More than half the time the call is not for a fire at all, but for a minor medical problem. In many cities, both fire trucks and ambulances respond to the same calls. This is not even close to an efficient way to deliver care. There are more rational systems to mimic. *Eastside Fire & Rescue* in Washington State, for one, operates a pilot program that eliminates fire trucks for most calls. They dispatch a single medic in an SUV first. In a majority of cases, that's all it takes. In the final analysis, it is entirely possible to improve outcomes by changing thinking. We can collectively create a new approach by the application of common sense.

Now if Code-3 driving is so often a mistake, why do we do it? Here is precisely why we do it:

Immutable Law #4

We love lights & sirens. They impress the public; They impress politicians; they impress us. They brandish the 'hurry up or else' sword by EMS authority over EMS personnel. They convince us we are more than episodically relevant.

"I don't know about you, but if I drop on the street observed or unobserved, I suppose somebody will feel obligated to call 911. But please do not administer CPR on me. I don't want my rib cage collapsed and I don't want to live with iatrogenic squash rot, only to have to die all over again sometime later."

—George Lundberg, MD, former Editor
Journal of the American Medical Association

Chapter Five

If CPR were an airline, who on earth would fly it?

In three plus decades of treating patients I can recall the faces of each person who lived to make it out of the hospital, after my partners and I performed CPR on them. That isn't because I've mastered Harry Lorayne's *Memory Power*. It's because there are only nine of them.

Nine, out of 1,102 resuscitation efforts. That's what I have to show for the gleeful aspect of my career called, "CPR saves." Happy to do the math for you: that's eight-tenths of 1%.

In spite of all the advancements and recent changes in protocols, the overall effectiveness of CPR remains depressingly low. Precise survival information is nearly impossible to quantify. The best most studies can show us is what happens in specific groups of people under specific circumstances during a given timeframe. Research done in 2012 indicates that fewer than 2% of adults who receive CPR in public places recover. Other studies have shown 4% and even higher, for patients who received CPR from bystanders and were eventually discharged from the hospital. Of course a regretful number are discharged to hospice facilities in multiple system failure. What no research has shown – because it may be impossible – is how many "survivors" actually had heartbeats all along, but simply fainted. Because the fact is, typical folks walking down the street would be hard pressed to find their own pulses, let alone the pulse of a stranger on a sidewalk next to a rumbling city bus, in an unexpected, highly stressful scenario where they feel expected to do something.

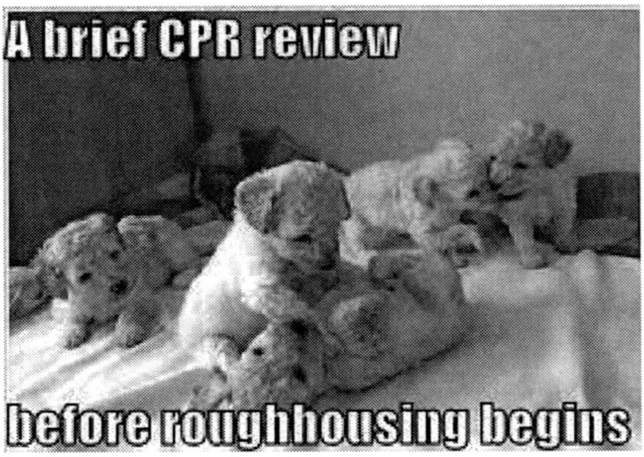

Are these little fellows any more naïve than we are?

It is a sad footnote to American society that the public has an almost childlike misconception about the effectiveness of CPR. And much of this is the direct result of television-created, cartoonish myths absorbed by non-thinking citizens. As far back as 15 years ago, a *Duke University* research team watched about 100 episodes of television medical dramas, such as ER and *Rescue 911.* They recorded the events of CPR during these shows – how it was administered and what results were depicted. What they discovered was a Hollyweird world where three out of every four patients lived after their hearts had "stopped." Some of them actually coughed a couple of times, grinned sheepishly and sat up to greet their saviors. Many of the shows were fiction, of course. But the CPR results were beyond science fiction. The only thing more outrageous than the drama is the fact that otherwise conscious adults believe such goofiness.

In the real world those fortunate few who successfully survive a heart-stopping event are what we call the "healthy dead," such as a person choking, where the airway can be cleared within minutes, or a child with a high fever, who can be cooled and resuscitated. Of course there are many more.

By far and away, the typical patients whose hearts stop beating are quite the opposite – the "unhealthy dead" – those who suffer from chronic illnesses, culminating in lethal systemic problems. These almost never survive. And they number 8,000 poor souls per day.

In their cases, pounding on their chests is, in our opinion, unnecessarily invasive and cruel, with practically no chance of benefit. Many "survivors" suffer pain they can no longer even tell us about, which must be about as close to hell on earth as there is.

A few years ago a Japanese study found that of 95,000 cases in which CPR had been performed in Japan in a single year, at the end of that year only 3% had what you would call a good outcome, a return to a meaningful quality of life. Another 3% wound up in a chronic vegetative state; 2% lingered in an in-between phase – not brain-dead, but not functional.

The remaining 92 % were dead.

"CPR is only useful when the heart stops because of a temporary problem that can be reversed or treated," says Doctor David Newman. Newman directs clinical research for the department of medicine at *Mount Sinai School of Medicine* in New York. He told the *Washington Post* that, "CPR was never meant for trauma like a car accident; never meant for those deathly ill. Cardiac arrest in too many scenarios is not a survivable condition. And even when we say it works, what we mean is that the hearts bounced back. Instead of dying then, they die later in ICU with the tubes and wires and pain and enormous expense for families."

CPR, he stresses, was never meant to be used at the end of long-term, chronic conditions.

"We've gotten confused about where CPR is good – almost a miracle – and where CPR is an abuse. What we too often do is unwanted by the patient. It is unduly invasive and burdensome to both provider and patient," Newman told the Post. "It should be done when theirs is a substantial chance of full recovery and the patient can safely be presumed to have wanted it."

But not in the netherworld of EMS, where the mandate is to do anything and everything to try to revive these poor people, unless a specific 'do not resuscitate' form is present.

Over the years we've been fortunate enough to know and work with hundreds of physicians. As early as 1979 we were taking notes on their answers to this simple question: "When the time comes, do you want CPR performed on *you*?"

We have always found their responses as revealing as anything in the wide world of health care. Not a single physician – out of 300+ who have been asked – not a single one, has ever answered "Yes."

Invariably, doctors say a big fat "No" to the same resuscitation efforts that he or she administers to their patients. Retired physician Ken Murray published an excellent article on just this subject in *The Guardian* in 2012, entitled *"How Doctors Choose to Die."*

You might want to look it up.

Murray noted that after decades of witnessing and administering medical care that makes people suffer, many doctors diagnosed with terminal illnesses choose to spend their last months or years at home and without medical treatment. They say "absolutely not" to major surgeries; they turn down chemotherapy and radiation for cancers. Murray reports that some of his colleagues have actually gotten tattoos that read, "No Code" to advise rescuers to not even think about starting chest compressions.

Physicians die too, you know. But few die in the same way their patients do. What makes a world of difference between the deaths of doctors and deaths of their patients is the sheer amount of medical treatment they choose to avoid. After investing decades doing battle with the wicked ailments of others, they know the routine. They can generally avail themselves to the most 'successful' treatments known to man. But guess what? They almost never do.

It isn't that physicians look forward to leaving this earth. Most are highly motivated to continue on. But they comprehend the limitations of modern medicine, even while they have been outwardly denying it their entire careers. So they lay the foundation of their demise beforehand. When their time comes, there will be no "heroics" on them. The last sensation they experience will assuredly not be a 200 pound first-aid zealot cracking their ribcage and buying them hours or days or weeks of hell on earth.

One need not be a physician to have seen what we all call, "futile care." Assaulted by needles; perforated by lances; strangled by tubes and doped by drugs. All of this starts with Paramedics; continues into the ER and – if you're lucky – extends for weeks in an ICU at a jaw-dropping cost of tens of thousands of dollars per day.

What it buys is misery we would not inflict on a terrorist.

Physicians know too well that the common outcomes of chest compressions look like this: rib fractures, sternum fractures, bleeding in the chest cavity, bleeding in the sac surrounding the heart and heart bruising.

So what do doctors want done on themselves?

Oh, there's more: airway damage; tearing the abdominal viscus; lacerations to the liver or spleen; fat emboli; lung bruising and lung tearing and lung bleeding.

To which the highest medically educated on the planet say "no thanks."

Doctor Murray still supports the efforts to teach the public CPR, because there are excellent instances when the emergency can be solved. But he also thinks it's time for the fresh air of realism when it comes to citizen training.

"People have too high expectations about what's going to happen," he said. "They think you're going to do CPR and the patient will eventually wake up. That's just not the case."

One confounding aspect is that so many in EMS mistake all medical treatment for health care. What the patients often need isn't 'treatment' at all, but guidance on how to talk with their physicians and family members to guarantee that death will happen on their terms, which in many cases would not include

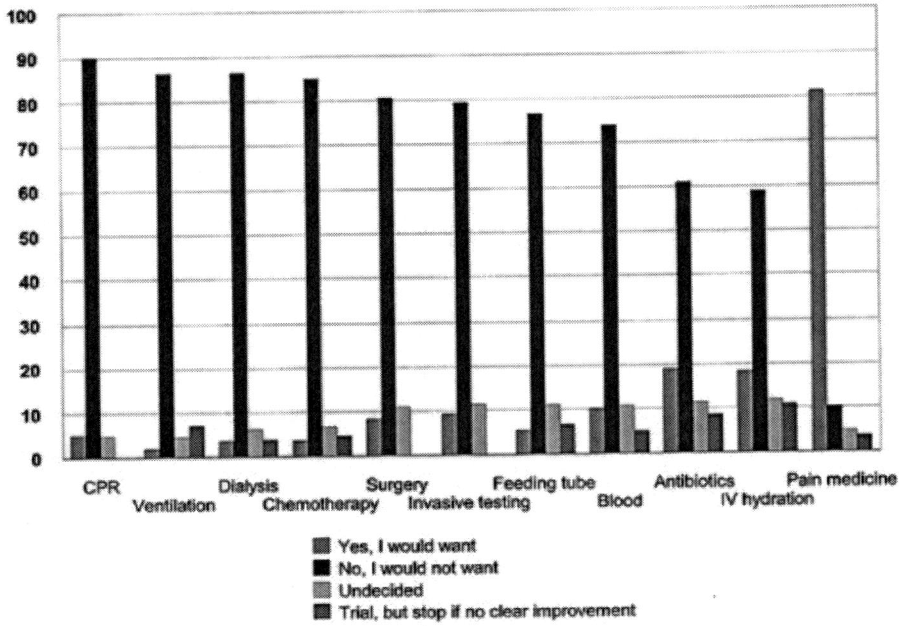

the violence of chest compressions, followed by an ICU imprisonment, tethered to mechanical devices they've never even heard of. In countless thousands of cases each year, if people simply understood how to manage the matter of their own deaths, EMS would not be called, and the 911 system could focus on getting appropriate responses to those who might actually benefit.

❖

Sometimes death is a foregone conclusion. And when that happens Paramedics follow a Death Scene Protocol that looks like this:

Victims who appear to have expired will not be resuscitated or transported by EMS personnel if obvious signs of death are present:

The four presumptive signs of clinical death are:

- No pulse
- No respirations
- Non-responsive
- Fixed & dilated pupils

Resuscitation must be initiated on all of the above cases, unless one of the following is also present:

The obvious signs of biological death are:

- Body decomposition
- Decapitation
- Corporal transection
- Incineration
- Rigor mortis
- Dependent lividity
- Massive or crushing trauma to the head or neck
- Avulsion of the brain or abdominal organs
- Submersion bloating

If there is any doubt regarding patient viability, resuscitation will be initiated.

When it is determined that the patient has expired and resuscitation will not be attempted, immediately notify the appropriate authority. DO NOT leave a body unattended DO NOT remove any property from the body or the scene for any reason NEVER transport/move a body except in consultation with the Coroner's office.

If the body is in public and cannot be blocked from view, it may be covered with a sterile Body Sheet.

❖

Plenty of medics remember their first CPR on a human being and I can recall mine with some detail. I was a freshly-minted EMT working in the California desert community of El Centro three decades ago. My partner was an EMT veteran who told me the first day I met him exactly why he had flunked out of Paramedic training: he just couldn't master EKGs. But he was an excellent ambulance man and a great partner and I was learning from him every day. And I think it was our third shift together when the call came in as a "man down . . . CPR in progress."

About 10 minutes later we turned into a neighborhood where a dozen people stood in the street frantically waving us toward a house. We grabbed our equipment and followed them around to the backyard, where we could see a lot of activity gathered around a low, metal-framed cot. It was a cool February afternoon. The narrow bed was situated in the shade beneath a large tree. Somebody was performing chest compressions on the man lying there, and with each deep thrust the old bed springs would sink him nearly to the ground. Everyone called him "uncle" and a woman told us he was 58 years old. As far as they knew he was on no medications. The pronounced capillary spidering across his face told us he was a severe alcoholic. We took over the scene and carefully dragged the fellow off the bed and onto the lawn.

From that point on J.B. Brown and I went into automatic mode. I cannot remember the ambulance ride to the ER. The next thing I knew we were rolling the gurney through the automatic doors of *El Centro Community Hospital*. With a group synchronized, "1, 2, 3, lift," we got our patient onto a hospital bed. The ER doctor on duty was Ed Iliff – one of the coolest young MDs we ever worked around. He removed the oral airway we'd placed into the patient's mouth and intubated the fellow within seconds. He then looked over at us as the nurses worked around him and asked, "How long has this gentleman been down?"

J.B. glanced at his watch and said, "At least 30 minutes."

Ed Iliff stopped what he was doing and turned toward the clock on the wall. He looked at the ER head nurse. "Let's call it right now, Gail. Time of death, 4:55."

And that was it.

I recall standing in the men's room splashing cold water in my face. When somebody's heart stops it can cause your own to beat a little harder. I could sense mine returning to normal. Even in the best case scenarios, resuscitation is serious effort – physically and emotionally draining. But the entire event bothered me because I'd thought we had done everything right.

Later that evening over dinner, I asked my partner for a critique of our service to the poor fellow. J.B. peered at me through his dark-rimmed glasses. "We did just fine. For your first outing you did great. I'm not remembering any mistakes or delays at all."

"But the guy died."

"Of course he died."

I'm sure I looked confused. "So if we'd gotten there earlier or . . . ."

"It might have helped," he answered quickly. "We don't know how long he was out on that bed. The family said he was taking his usual nap under the tree. Nobody knows when he stopped breathing."

I nodded slowly. "So, how many of these things have you been on?"

He gazed up at the ceiling for an answer. "I don't know. We get two or three a month and I've been doing this for three years. Quite a few."

"Do they usually live?"

"No, they pretty much never live. I think the medics had a save last year, but it started as an airway obstruction, so the patient didn't really have a heart problem. Kids can bounce back because it isn't usually heart-related at all. They've got perfect little pumps and perfect little pipes. When it comes to CPR saves, the younger they are the better. But people over 50? Don't count on it."

Don't count on it?

Fast forward to five years later. I was employed by *Medevac, Incorporated* in San Diego, the fastest growing EMS provider in the nation. We had a *UCSD* med school education and the finest equipment money could buy. We had great teamwork, outstanding fire support and pretty quick response times. We had 14 ERs to take our patients to. The medics in our city were running 108 CPR cases a month. How many were we saving?

Maybe one. On a good month . . . three.

Wait a minute. Grab your guppies. Let's clarify something important. It all depends on what you mean by "save." The semantics of medicine can drive a sane person nuts, and one of our favorite little flapdoodles is called a "field save." A perfect example of a field save is when medics arrive to find a patient with, for example, a highly irregular heart rhythm, one that cannot generate enough circulation to keep you alive for very long. Let's say we get there and your blood pressure – which normally might be, maybe 138/86 – is now 50/30. For an adult such a pressure is lethal – far too low to provide adequate nourishment to your major organs. So we hook you up to our portable EKG and determine your kooky heart rhythm is the cause of the problem. We start an IV line; inject a drug that smoothes out your irregular heartbeat. Just for fun, we'll call the drug xylocaine. We mix a follow-up dose in a bag of fluid that drips slowly into your arm and keeps you on an even keel. We put you on oxygen, get your blood pressure up to 120/90 and take you to the ER. Two hours later you die of a massive pulmonary embolism. That's a fancy term for a clot of blood or fat in your lungs.

If this patient were your mother, would you consider her life saved? Would you be pleased? Would you bake us a 'thank you cake?' No? Why not?

We would be pleased. Paramedics would be downright gleeful.

The fact that she died doesn't mean we didn't save her. You just think we didn't save her. But we know we did. Her blood pressure was dangerously low when we got to her and normal when we got her to the ER. We reached into our nifty bag of tricks; interpreted her EKG as well as any cardiologist; pushed some serious drugs (our favorite thing in the whole wide world to do, by the way) and pulled out a viable circulation. Ergo, we 'saved her.' Get it?

I personally have handled countless cases just like this. I reached the point where I was actually unzipped enough to enjoy the accolades for the 'save' on the same day as the funeral. Medicine is chock full of mind-twisted little jargogles. And the nurses' congratulatory hugs aren't bad either. It is amazing how many romances get started as the result of CPR 'saves' when the patients get buried. Those hugs go a long, long way toward tamping down our group-think EMS dementia.

Are you listening? We don't call it the *Twilight Zone* for nothing.

Immutable Law #5

We do CPR because it makes us feel useful. We consider it dress-rehearsal for other people. We do it because hopeless chest compressions rake in billions.

"The International Classification of Diseases, 10th revision (known as the ICD-10) identifies 69,823 diagnoses – 69,823 maladies you just might have. We're chomping at the bit that you have at least one, because we have 71,924 different things we can do to you, and 3,700 different drugs we can pop into your mouth or squirt into your veins. What could possibly go wrong?"

—The Author

Chapter Six

You say you want to go to the hospital?
You seem like a nice person, so let's
see if we can't talk you out of that.

Now that you recognize health care swims in Ironic River, you are in the perfect frame of mind to appreciate this little pickle: the single most dangerous place you will ever find yourself is in a hospital.

❖

"Anyone who understands systems will know immediately that optimizing parts is not a good route to system excellence. You've heard I'm sure of the famous experiment when they tried to build the world's greatest car by assembling the world's greatest car parts. They connected the engine of a Ferrari; the brakes of a Porsche; the suspension of a BMW; the body of a Volvo. What they created was nothing close to a great car. What they got was a pile of very expensive junk. In medicine, that is exactly what we have done."
Doctor Donald Berwick
President, Institute for Healthcare Improvement

❖

Want us to wait while you go pour yourself a nice, soothing drink? For the first time in its highly respectable history, *Consumer Reports* has weighed in, turning a non-medical eye onto the subject of hospital safety. For decades they've been opening our eyes to crashing cars and testy toasters. More than 170 other studies have been done, of course – nearly all by medical folks and therefore tweaked toward partisan. But *Consumer Reports* owns a terrific history of objectivity and frankly, they don't care whether we like them or not. They do not bother expressing politically correct findings. So if their stuff doesn't frighten you, maybe you are already dead and don't know it.

Consumer Reports operates a fairly recent program they refer to as the Health Ratings Center, which brings focus upon six sub-categories of concern:

- Death rates
- Clinical safety communications
- Side effects and complications
- Radiation caused by too many imaging tests
- Hospital-acquired infections
- Re-admissions after patients have been told they are well enough to go home

The number of poorly performing hospitals their research uncovered is alarming in itself. But the severity and volume of the resulting harm to the citizens of this country – the direct result of medically miscreant ways – is nothing short of jaw-dropping.

❖

"If medical error were a recognized disease category, it would be the leading cause of death in the United States."
Doctor Carolyn Dean, Medical Researcher

❖

Unlike *U.S. News & World Report* – which churns out its highly touted 'Best Hospital' list each year with the chimerical fancy of a teenage girl at a rock concert – *Consumer Reports* does not allow itself to go gaga over a hospital's glossy reputation. Reputation is prestige and too often is the PR result of clinical success of highly technical surgical procedures. Prestige makes headlines. The reality is, almost none of us will ever need a liver transplant. Few will shop for a face replacement. (Although we wouldn't mind seeing our options) Choosing a hospital based on such criteria can put you and your family into deep doo-doo. So don't do that.

Remember as you lie in bed awaiting your appendix removal, keep in mind that your chances of a urinary tract infection from a hospital cootie is of considerable more relevance, than is that patient down the hallway with the successful heart transplant.

Of course most patients don't choose their hospital at all. Rather, they go where their doctors happen to have staff privileges. That is called "luck." And we can promise you that physicians can be just as ignorant about hospital safety as their patients are. Sometimes more so, since as a patient you have a lot more down time to actually look around.

This study found that even the so-called 'best' hospitals are not performing as well as they think they are, nor as well as many smaller community clinics with considerably less money to spend on patient safety. One major reason for this is that too many larger, 'famous' medical centers simply see no reason to change very much. In fact, some of the best-known teaching hospitals do not rank very high, either.

The top-rated teaching hospitals, which train physicians, were found to be these. Keep in mind a perfect score is 100%, just like high school:

68% - *The Mayo Clinics* in Rochester, Minnesota, Phoenix & Jacksonville
66% - *Gundersen Medical Center*, La Crosse Wisconsin
65% - *Bronson Methodist,* Kalamazoo Michigan
65% - *St. Mary's Hospital,* Waterbury Connecticut
64% - *Ball Memorial Hospital,* Muncie Indiana

63% - *Avera McKennan*, Sioux Falls South Dakota
63% - *Baystate Medical Center*, Springfield Massachusetts
62% - *University of Utah,* Salt Lake City
The lowest rated teaching hospitals are:
30% - *Saint Louis University Hospital*, Saint Louis
30% - *University Medical Center*, Lubbock Texas
29% - *Jacobi Medical Center,* New York
28% - *Harlem Hospital,* New York
28% - *Westchester Medical Center,* New York
28% - *Tulane Medical Center,* New Orleans
27% - *Shands Medical Center,* Jacksonville

An embarrassing 33% of the nation's teaching hospitals – you know, where doctors are born – score above average. Of the 258 total, 172 are below average. In the New York area, **Winthrop University Medical Center** in Mineola – no, not *Sloan-Kettering* nor *Presbyterian* – was the only one of 28 teaching hospitals to be rated higher than mediocre.

If there is anything more educational in these findings, it might be that fewer than 30% of this country's 5,800+ clinical providers volunteered to respond to the study in the first place. And of those who did respond, the nationwide mean rating was 49%.

Of course, if we thought we'd score as low as the dunce-cap crowd, we might not respond to a publicly exposed research request either. Maybe you remember how a bright red "F" looked at the top of a quiz page when you were in high school. Hopefully it wasn't yours.

So if you are looking for good news about patient safety, we recommend you just visit your local hospital's website and enjoy their flashy PR. Trust us: there is no chance at all they will depress you even a little bit, by letting on how many people died under their roof unnecessarily last year.

❖

"It is impossible to justify the fact that thousands of hospitals, which collectively have granted admitting privileges to

hundreds of thousands of doctors, have not reported a single physician discipline case in 17 years."
Doctor Sidney Wolfe, Public Citizen
Co-founder, Health Research Group

❖

How could hospitals be so dangerous?

Well before *Consumer Report* pulled the curtain on dream world, an eye-opening study by the *Institute of Medicine* 13 years ago uncovered that 100,000 people were dying every year as the direct result of medical error. And thousands of these folks trusted Paramedics to take them to a safe place.

Ironic, isn't it?

In spite of medical advances since that study – or in many cases because of them – a recent update shows that the actual number of people who die because of medical error is closer to 250,000 per year. Happy to do the math for you: that's 685 souls every 24 hours. You would have to crash three airliners every day of the month to equal that kind of carnage. In a mind-numbing *Health Affairs* review in 2011, their study revealed that medical errors happen to one of every three patients hospitalized overnight. So you have a busy hospital in your town with 300 beds? Good for you. Now quick, before you blink: how many occupants of those beds can expect to come down with an avoidable complication by tomorrow? We can wait while you do the math . . . .

An entirely separate assessment of folks on Medicare determined that one patient in seven suffers at least one malady that prolongs their stay; causes permanent injury; requires life-sustaining treatment, or kills them.

And finally, in a telephone survey of the American public, 33 out of every 100 reported personal experiences with medical error, and 50% stated that a relative was the victim of a medical mistake. Many happened in out-patient clinics, of course. Plenty of others happened in doctors' offices. But nearly all happened in hospitals.

❖

"There is an epidemic of health-care harm. More than 2,225,000 Americans will probably die from medical injury in this decade. That's like wiping out the entire populations of North Dakota, Rhode Island and Vermont. It's a man-made disaster. And we all just keep pretending it isn't happening."
Rosemary Gibson, patient safety advocate
Author, the Wall of Silence

❖

We don't know what you choose for bedtime reading but we like things like this:

July spike in fatal medication errors: a possible effect of new medical residents
Phillips, DP; Barker GE

Source
Department of Sociology, University of California at San Diego, 0533, 9500 Gilman Drive, La Jolla, CA 92093-0533, USA. dphillips@ucsd.edu

Background
Each July thousands begin medical residencies and acquire increased responsibility for patient care. Many have suggested that these new medical residents may produce errors and worsen patient outcomes-the so-called "July Effect;" However, we have found no U.S. evidence documenting this effect.

Objective
Determine whether fatal medication errors spike in July.

Design
We examined all U.S. death certificates, 1979-2006 (n = 62,338,584), focusing on medication errors (n = 244,388). We compared the observed number of deaths in July with the number expected, determined by least-squares regression techniques. We

compared the July Effect inside versus outside medical institutions. We also compared the July Effect in counties with versus without teaching hospitals.

Outcome Measure
JR = Observed number of July deaths / Expected number of July deaths.

Results
Inside medical institutions, in counties containing teaching hospitals, fatal medication errors spiked by 10% in July and in no other month [JR = 1.10 (1.06-1.14)]. In contrast, there was no July spike in counties without teaching hospitals. The greater the concentration of teaching hospitals in a region, the greater the July spike (r = .80; P = .005). These findings held only for medication errors, not for other causes of death.

Here's their conclusion:
We found a significant July spike in fatal medication errors inside medical institutions. After assessing competing explanations, **we concluded that the July mortality spike results at least partly from changes associated with the arrival of new medical residents.**

Well that certainly lends itself to a restful sleep.

❖

Health care likes to pretend that it creates health. If you believe that, you might also believe that Einstein created the law of relativity and the world experienced no gravity before Newton. Everybody just . . . floated around.

❖

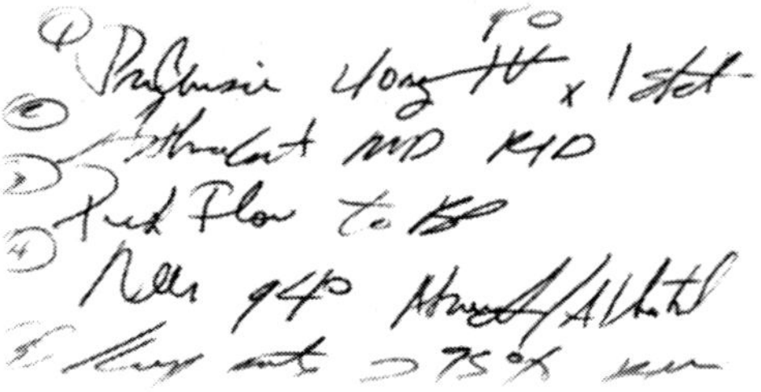

How often have YOU played prescription pad Russian roulette?

As interns we were thrilled that the exciting drugs we were squirting into you people were grounded in evidence – preternatural end-products of impartial testing and clinical trials. After all, one of our perplexing secrets is that the societal value we Paramedics place in ourselves, lies in direct proportion to how many drugs we are legally allowed to push. So we inject gallons of dubious magic into thousands of folks before we learn those tests and trials are often sinfully flawed. When you start out as a medic you reckon that MDs who issue medication orders over the telephone are well-versed in the drug research literature. It is depressing that so many of my colleagues never bother to learn that much of the research is hidden from all of us, by the pharmaceutical juggernauts. In the *Twilight Zone* this is not even a matter of discussion during medic down-time, even as we witness countless drug-related death scenes. That's called whistling past the graveyard.

I once actually imagined that physicians were impartially educated. Then I discovered that much of their education is funded by drug cartels. Like so many others, I presumed the *FDA* operated under a rigid code of ethics that would only permit safe and effective drugs to be prescribed by the cartels. It is a slap in the face of our profession that the *FDA* has a long history of approving worthless and dangerous drugs, knowing full well that data on side effects are routinely withheld by the drug makers who have been fined billions for lying. I now know that blind faith in medicine holds all the trappings of a neurological disorder. It abdicates your wellbeing to those who profit from your ill-being. Consider this fact for a mere 10 seconds, please:

we actually accept that mass death is a normal by-product of what we do.

❖

Imagine you are sitting on a modern airliner, waiting for the jet to head out toward the runway to leap into the air above our heads. You're looking forward to that big bag of pretzels. You gaze out the window to see the pilot and co-pilot come rushing up the stairs and into the cockpit. Within a few seconds the pilot's voice comes over the intercom, advising the passengers, "Ladies and gentlemen, please fasten your seatbelts. We're ready for takeoff."

Can you think of any critical little matter that ought to have happened but didn't? Like, did they have time for a safety check? No, no safety check was performed. You know, doors locked? Check. Wheel chocks removed? Check. Engines synchronized? Check. Do we have enough gas . . . .

Checklists – in addition to brutally transparent incident reports – have helped transform aviation from one of the most lethal activities humans could do, into the safest manner of transportation on the planet. Last year there was not a single fatal airliner crash on the continent. The fatal incident rate of 1:2,500,000 flights made 2012 the safest year in the history of aviation.

From manned flight to shipbuilding to Tinker Toys, checklists and public reporting of abnormal incidents have become an integral part of safety improvement in practically every challenging human activity. And the key word here is 'transparency.' But in health care? Hey. Who are you to tell us what to do? The world of medicine lags far behind other complex endeavors when it comes to safety improvement, or in letting anybody know who the spooks are. And we really dislike outsiders knowing, else they start snooping around in things that are none of your business, like why aunt Martha really died.

Underscoring this fact is a report from the *Department of Health and Human Services* last year, which revealed that of any given seven patients harmed in a hospital, merely one is ever reported. Why blab about the bad stuff? The Inspector General estimates that the true rate of Medicare patients suffering 'adverse events' is 10,000 per week. And that's just the elderly.

Hospital administrators have had plenty of time to focus on this ugliness, and some medical centers have made great strides in reducing errors and infections by using – hold your ponies – checklists.

We're impressed. It only took them 150 years.

Today there are dozens of checklists for many of the trickiest procedures. Doctor Atul Gawande even wrote a best-selling book about the value of checklists in medicine: *The Checklist Manifesto.* So do you think by now every hospital in the country operates under mandated checklist protocols?

Don't be ridiculous.

❖

American healthcare: the best in the world?

Well, we know the fantasy you probably cling to like a Teddy Bear. But before you say it out loud, take a look at what Doctor Barbara Starfield of *Johns Hopkins School of Public Health* told the world on July 26, 2000, in the *Journal of the American Medical Association*, when she reported what was happening **each year**:

- 7,000 people dying from medication errors in hospitals
- 12,000 people dying from unnecessary surgeries
- 20,000 people dying from other errors in hospitals
- 80,000 people dying from infections acquired in hospitals
- 106,000 people dying from prescription medications

Care to guess what your local EMS men and women have to say about this jaw-dropping reality? Nothing. The quietest people in town when it comes to bad medicine – even quieter than nurses – are Paramedics. Our comfort meters function best in the nether-world of, "why risk my job?"

So guess what? We don't.

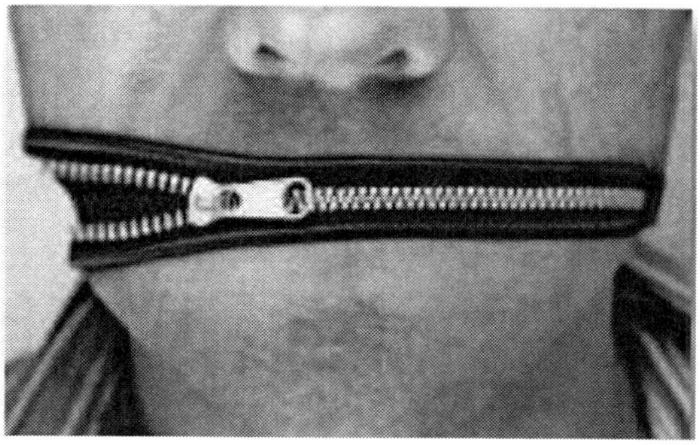

Typical Paramedic reaction to bad doctoring

Wimpy reaction, comrades. The correct response is that you – we – are medical professionals bright enough to recognize horse shit when we see it. Take a stance; open your mouths and speak up. Dashing out the door to stop the bleeding is not the only way to save lives. Remember the admonition at the beginning of this book:

"Make no mistake. Medicine has always engendered a fertile ground for capitalistic predators. It provides terrific niches for off-the-chart sociopaths. And too many of us who are not, have become ingeniously adept at hiding those who are. Paramedics are particularly guilty."

The ugly truth is some of the most macho medics on the planet turn into complete lollipops in the presence of an arrogant, incompetent physician. And that, amigos, is little more than Paramedic poltroonery.

So Doctor Barbara Starfield's conclusion? The estimated number of deaths caused by medical treatment in America was at that time 225,000 each year. Imagine if you woke up tomorrow to read that somebody poisoned the water in Lincoln, Nebraska and today every resident is now dead. Or Orlando, Florida. How about Reno, Nevada.

The mind-numbing reality? Our medical system was the third-leading cause of death – right after heart disease and cancer – 12 years ago.

But surely we've learned our lessons since then, right?

Doctor Carolyn Dean, author of *Death by Modern Medicine: Seeking Safer Solutions* would say absolutely not. Her study found that 11 common medical mistakes killed 900,000 patients in 2008. Lord have mercy. It revealed that an estimated

15,000,000 Americans – out of 37,000,000 patients who were admitted – suffer medical harm in hospitals, every year. Outside of this jaw-dropping human toll, medical errors cost the health-care system $17,100,000,000 every 12 months.

You might want to go back and ogle all those zeros.

But what does this all mean? It means that in a court of law, U.S. health care would have the Devil's own time convincing a jury with the collective IQ of a gerbil, that it saves more people than it kills.

And personally? We no longer have faith that it would win that argument.

Keep in mind too, these numbers are not disputed. To the contrary. Over the past dozen years, follow-up researchers have found the number of preventable deaths due to medical intervention is higher. A lot higher.

So why on earth wouldn't every hospital be clambering toward safety and away from patient danger? Well friends, there's a ton of money in screw-ups.

❖

Hospitals making money on their own mistakes?

Here in the *Twilight Zone* there is very little profit in safety and not much more in good health. There is, however, utter wealth in medical complications. In all four corners of bizarre world, substandard care is rewarded with serious cash in return. For those of a grab-thy-money mindset, it really doesn't get much better than this. And when the rampallians wear lab coats, they can fool themselves – and most everybody else – by acting as though whatever they choose to do is probably right. A Sunday afternoon visit to a cemetery is proof enough that unseeing faith in medicine has rather sobering limitations.

Fee-for-service works just fine when discussing roof repairs and lawn care. But for medical corporations and physicians to get paid for each service they provide – with no bearing on whether it is necessary or properly done – is beyond foolish for society to tolerate. Fee for service guarantees that the poor will receive only a fraction of care that they desperately need. It absolutely promises that people with money will get far more "care" than they should sit still for. The entire conundrum seeds the fertile garden of altruism with a nearly impossible-to-avoid temptation. It creates perverse environments where true wealth can be amassed by additional services, which neither the payer nor the patient are in any real position to valuate.

❖

"We could improve dismal health outcomes on both ends of the socio-economic spectrum if we were simply faithful to science; if we provided and practiced care we knew to be effective."
Otis Webb Brawley, MD
Chief Medical Officer, American Cancer Society

❖

Consider that a hospital can net a typical $18,000 profit for a flawless operation. But did you know they can rake in $50,000 for that same surgery, if there are complications or mistakes needing further treatment? Complications and errors double the profit if the patient is insured by Medicare. And the profit triples when the patient has private insurance.

Are you starting to sense our ire here?

One excellent study used a measure of profit called the 'contribution margin' and found that surgical missteps and complications involving the heart, peripheral nerve tracks and spinal chord are a boon to the bottom line. Researchers studied 34,000 surgical records and discovered consistent trends.

Doctor Barry Rosenberg, Managing Director of the *Boston Consulting Group*, which did the research, sums it up very clearly:

"If a patient has colon cancer surgery, Medicare pays a certain fee. But if that patient gets a post-operative infection that leads to pneumonia and has to be put on a ventilator for several days, the payment for ventilator care is far higher and more profitable than the payment for the original surgery."

❖

Common hospital complications

If you expect to be hospitalized overnight you should know that these preventable drawbacks should keep you and your family particularly vigilant:

Surgical Errors:

In all 50 states, one of the most lethal things that can happen to you is a surgical error. Operation on the wrong patient; operation on the right patient but the wrong body part; sometimes the right body part on the right patient but the wrong procedure; or maybe the right procedure performed badly. If you can take a *Johns Hopkins University* study at its word, these happen 4,000 times a year. But keep in mind, these are just the ones that are reported, and one particular category – patients catching on fire – is notorious for never being reported at all. Who wants to admit they flash-cooked grandpa?

Hospital-acquired Infections:

By this point in the evolution of society the term 'nosocomial infection' should be a household phrase. The fact that even our computer's spell-check fails to recognize the term, tells us all we need to know about the utterly relentless juggernaut called health care advertizing. After all, anything that can kill 4,000 citizens a week without making *Eyewitness News* knows how to cover its tracks. Incidentally, *Resources for the Future*, a non-profit research group, came up with that number.

Medication Errors:

The most common prescription errors happen when a drug is given at the wrong time; or to the wrong patient; or in the wrong dose. How often does it happen badly enough to kill people? Well, according to *HealthGrades*' Patient Safety Study, drug mistakes kill 3,200 patients every week of the year. And remember, this is the medical system that wants to outlaw vitamins, because every now and then, somebody gets a tummy ache.

Blood Clots:

Because of inactivity during a hospital stay, your circulation is reduced and blood in the veins tends to clot. A clot can become lodged in the deep blood vessels, which is a condition called deep vein thrombosis (DVT). When a clot breaks free, it can travel through your blood stream and block the blood flow in narrow passageways of your lungs. This is called a pulmonary embolus (PE). These conditions kill thousands of people every year.

Bedsores:

Actually they are more properly called pressure ulcers: a breakdown of skin that results from lying in one position too long. This pressure on a foot, a hip, a shoulder, cuts off circulation to the area. They can become infected and the infection can burrow deep into bones and joints. If the bacteria get into your bloodstream you can develop sepsis, which is very dangerous.

❖

From day one of training we learn to parrot that we are about to become key components to the "finest health care system in the world." And like the talking birds around me, I got so accustomed to hearing it that I vapidly figured it was probably true. Why was it true? Well, because people in lab coats kept saying it was true. And in the movies, if you wear white, you've got to be one of the good guys. Get it?

The problem is, it was not true. It was not true 30 years ago and it surely is not true today. Here is a more enlightened way to look at it, so please do:

The 'best' of American health care is as fine and dandy as any. No question. The typical U.S. health care is far better than that which most of the other 195 nations can offer. But 'most' means simply outshining 98 other countries. We have a long, long way to go, to compete with the top three-dozen on earth. Care to see how we compare to 10 European nations and Canada?

World healthcare rankings (1st-37th)

- ***1st in Health Care Costs*** - $2.6 trillion, $8,000 a year per person
- ***1st in Obesity*** – 33% of adult citizens are obese. In 1980 it was 15%

- ***2nd in Diabetes*** – 10% of us suffer from diabetes, surpassed only by Mexico's'11%. European average is 6%
- ***4th in Preventing Death from Stroke***
- ***7th in Cancer Frequency*** – Cancer strikes 300 of us per 100,000
- ***10th in Number Nurses*** – 10 per 1,000 people
- ***25th in Heart Disease Prevention*** – 129 deaths per 100,000 people
- ***27th in Life Expectancy*** – Americans can expect to live 78.2 years, below the European average and just behind Slovenia and Chile.
- ***30th in Hospital Beds available*** – per 1,000 population
- ***31st in Health Coverage*** – 4th from last, behind the Slovak Republic; 25 OECD countries cover 99% or more of their citizens.
- ***31st in Infant Mortality*** – .5 babies die per 1,000 live births
- ***31st in Preventing Premature Death*** – U.S. premature death is surpassed only by Hungary, Mexico and Russia – accidents, violence, cancer, circulatory disease.

Frankly we find this embarrassing. Across 14 categories of care, here is precisely how we stack up with those who are truly at the top of the food chain:

- France
- Italy
- San Marino
- Andorra
- Malta
- Singapore
- Spain
- Oman
- Austria
- Japan
- Norway
- Portugal

- Belgium
- Columbia
- Sweden
- Cyprus
- Germany
- Saudi Arabia
- United Arab Emirates
- Israel
- Morocco
- Canada
- Finland
- Australia
- Chile
- Denmark
- Dominica
- Costa Rica
- **United States**

This ranking was performed by the *World Health Organization.*

❖

Are you sure you want that operation?

Across this nation at least 3,000 people underwent unnecessary surgery today. Another 3,000 will be cut upon tomorrow. Many of these folks will be gravely injured and some will die as the result of physician assaults that ought never have happened in the first place. Here are some of the most common unnecessary, extremely profitable operations you might face once we Good Samaritans tote your body gently into the ER:

Hysterectomy:

Well over 10,000 hysterectomies a week are inflicted upon women of America, even though five studies have proven that most of them are not needed. Removal of the uterus is essential for long-term health when it is cancerous, but the fact is, that is only true in 10% of the cases. By far most women undergo the operation for no better reason than uterine fibroids – painful and bleeding, yes. Fibroids are abnormal but non-lethal growths in the uterine wall. But there are choices besides removal of the uterus. Women who undergo total hysterectomies face a higher risk of heart disease, lung cancer and urinary incontinence by age 60. If your physician does not at least discuss alternatives, such as focused ultrasound and uterine blood vessel embolization for fibroids, as well as laparoscopic – as opposed to vaginal – access, we strongly suggest you put your clothes back on and walk out the door.

Knee Arthroscopy for Osteoarthritis:

Arthroscopic knee surgery is the procedure of inserting a micro-camera through a hole past the skin tissue and into the joint – then working with small instruments through other incisions to repair damaged cartilage which supports the joint. Research has proven that this procedure is excellent in repairing torn meniscus ligaments with far less surrounding tissue injury than the old way of literally opening up the entire knee. But research also tells us arthroscopic surgery is not a better way to treat osteoarthritis. In studies which began in 2008, for example, osteoarthritis patients who were treated with non-invasive remedies reported better mobility with less pain and stiffness, than those who had the operation. Again, these options should be seriously discussed before anybody starts cutting on you.

Spinal Fusion for Stenosis:

This operation is frequently done to relieve pain caused by a condition called stenosis, which is what can happen over years when shock absorbing tissue between the bony vertebrae becomes worn down. Stenosis causes pressure on the nerves or the spinal chord itself.

A surgical fusion means pieces of bone are used to 'weld' at least two vertebrae together and sometimes several, to keep them from pushing against each other and therefore pinching nerves. Fusion has become the favored option for thousands of surgeons. In a five-year study that began in 2002, 30,000

Medicare fusion cases were viewed. Over that period the procedure increased a jaw-dropping 1,400%.

The downside of having spinal fusion is impressive. Patients who undergo complex fusion are three times more likely to suffer dangerous complications than those who have less invasive surgery. Research shows more than half of all spinal fusion patients continue to have as much or more back pain than those who used physical therapy and movement modifications. According to Doctor Floyd Fowler, science advisor for the *Foundation for Informed Medical Decision Making (FIMDM)*, "After fusion, the vertebrae just above and below the fusion are forced into more movement than before, and this in itself causes other injury and other pain."

Heart Stents for Stable Angina:

A stent is a tiny mesh tube that is surgically inserted into a narrow blood vessel within the heart. In the emergent situation of heart tissue death or near-death, a stent can absolutely save your life. But the overwhelming numbers of stent placements in this country are not used in emergencies at all – but for a chronic heart condition. And when that condition is chest pain brought on by exertion or stress, known as stable angina, a stent does not outperform diet and lifestyle changes and/or effective medications called statins, according to a major *Veterans Affairs* study conducted as far back as seven years ago.

In spite of this reality, surgeons are implanting stents at the stunning rate of 8,000 each week for stable chest pain. According to Sanjay Kaul, MD, a heart specialist at *Cedars-Sinai in Los Angeles*, surgeons often insert stents during catheterization procedures in order to evaluate the condition of the arteries. But it is becoming increasingly obvious that catheterization should be done as a diagnostic test first, and stent placement – if needed at all – should be done as a second procedure. Unfortunately, few patients are ever aware of this, and they do not leave the catheterization lab until after the stent is already inside them.

"The reality is that 20% of patients who undergo this surgery do not have any symptoms at all. From 30% to 50% have not had a stress test, which they should, and 30% are not treated with medical therapy first," says Doctor Kaul. "If plaque is forming in your arteries, this is a systemic disease. A stent won't keep the rest of your arteries clear."

Outside the *Twilight Zone*, cutting people with sharp objects for profit is considered assault to commit bodily harm. Inside? We call it business as usual. Cue the weird music.

❖

Here is yet another curious reality:

The *Center for Disease Control* operates under the *Department of Health & Human Services.* The current *CDC* Director is Doctor Tom Frieden and this year 24 federal advisory committees exist. They provide advice and recommendations on a broad range of public health issues, to help the *CDC* achieve its mission, "to promote health and quality of life by preventing and controlling disease, injury, and disability." Among the program areas these committees address are occupational and environmental health; healthcare infection control; clinical laboratory standards; smoking; breast and cervical cancer; HIV, STDs and Tuberculosis; childhood and adult immunizations; and injury prevention and control. The key players at the *CDC* are:

<u>Advisory Committee to the Director</u>: Chairman: Alan Edward Greenberg MD, MPH; Professor Department of Epidemiology and Biostatistics, *George Washington University* School of Public Health

<u>Designated Federal Officer:</u> Carmen Villar MSW, Chief of Staff

<u>Members:</u>

Dileep G. Bal MD, District Health Officer, State of Hawaii

George C. Benjamin MD, Executive Director, *American Public Health Association*, Washington DC

Nisha D. Botchwey PhD, MPH, Professor, *Georgia Institute of Technology*
Benjamin K. Chu MD, MPH Group President, *Kaiser So. California & Hawaii*
Sylvia Drew Ivie JD, Exec. Liaison Commission, *Children & Families L.A.*

To your knowledge, has even one advisor on any *CDC* committee ever publicly addressed the fact that health care is a major cause of citizen death in the United States?

The answer is no.

Our question: why would an organization dedicated to national health – indeed, one which dutifully reports each year's "Top 10 Causes of Death" – refuse to acknowledge a category that kills hundreds of thousands? Errant health care kills 400 + citizens a day at least, yet the *CDC* has convinced an entire population to fret about the flu. At magic shows this is called 'misdirection.' Of course at magic shows, misdirection is usually a bellezeboobian in a skimpy costume. Different technique. Identical outcome.

The silence of the *CDC* regarding bad medicine is indefensible. And the silence of Paramedics – who can arguably stake claim as the truest lifesavers in town – is shameful.

Immutable Law #6

Errant health care kills more people than any single disease. In our world your death bothers us very little. It is acceptable collateral damage, because every now and then we do save somebody else.

"We call it 'buffing the charts' and around here we buff 'em till they shine."

—The Fat Man MD
The House of God

SERVICE NAME:
(PLEASE PRINT)

Patient Care Report

Service #:	Unit #:	Incident #: -	Pt. Record #:	Crash #:
Date of Onset: / /	Date Unit Notified: / /		Run Report Date: / /	Trauma ID #:

Dispatched For:

TIMES (MILITARY)			
Dispatch Notified:	: : :	Time Left Scene:	: : :
Unit Notified:	: : :	Arrived at Destination:	: : :
Unit Enroute:	: : :	Back In Service:	: : :
Arrived at Scene:	: : :	Total Incident Time:	: : :
Minutes For Response:	911 ☐ YES ☐ NO	Time of Injury/Illness:	
Minutes At Scene:			
Minutes For Transport:			

PATIENT INFORMATION

(Last Name) (First) (MI)

(Street Address) (Apt. #)

(City) (State) (Zip Code)

(Phone) (Date of Birth) (Age yrs. mons)

(Gender) ☐ M 1 ☐ F 2 ☐ Unk 3 (SSN#) __ __ __ - __ __ - __ __ __ __

Ethnicity ☐ 0 Other ☐ 1 Hispanic

Race ☐ 0 Other, including multi racial ☐ 1 White ☐ 2 Black ☐ 3 American Indian, Eskimo or Aleut ☐ 4 Asian ☐ U Undetermined

Chief Complaint:	Injury/Illness Narrative:
Past Medical History:	Pertinent Findings on Physical Exam:
Allergies:	Patient Medications:
Emerg. Med. Care Given:	Patient Response to Emerg. Med. Care:

Provider Impression: - Select one

☐ Abdominal Pain/Problems ☐ Airway Obstruction ☐ Alleged Sexual Assault ☐ Allergic Reaction ☐ Altered Level of Consciousness ☐ Behavioral Disorder ☐ Cardiac Arrest

☐ Cardiac Rhythm Disturbance ☐ Chest Pain/Discomfort ☐ Diabetic Symptoms ☐ Electrocution ☐ Hyperthermia ☐ Hypoglycemia ☐ Hypothermia (Disease)

☐ Hypothermia (Trauma) ☐ Hypovolemia ☐ Inhalation Injury (Toxic Gas) ☐ **Not Applicable** ☐ Obvious Death ☐ Other ☐ Poisoning/Drug Ingestion

☐ Pregnancy/OB Delivery ☐ Psychiatric Disorder ☐ Respiratory Arrest ☐ Respiratory Distress ☐ Seizure ☐ Shock ☐ Smoke Inhalation

☐ Stings/Venomous Bites ☐ Stroke/CVA ☐ Syncope/Fainting ☐ Traumatic Hypovolemia ☐ Traumatic Injury ☐ Vaginal Hemorrhage ☐ Unknown

Mutual Aid	EMS Tier	Destination / Transferred To	MODE OF TRANSPORT
			☐ Fixed Wing ☐ Ground ☐ **None** ☐ Other ☐ Rotor Craft

DESTINATION DETERMINATION/OUT OF HOSPITAL TRIAGE CRITERIA

☐ Closest Facility ☐ Diversion ☐ Family Choice ☐ Law Enforcement Choice

☐ Managed Care ☐ **Not Applicable** ☐ On-Line Medical Direction

☐ Other ☐ Patient Choice ☐ Patient Physician Choice

☐ Protocol ☐ Specialty Resource Center ☐ Trauma Triage (Anatomy of Injury)

☐ Trauma Triage (GCS, Vitals) ☐ Trauma Triage (Mechanism of Injury) ☐ Trauma Triage (Risk Factors) ☐ Unknown

CLINICAL INFORMATION

Time	B/P	PULSE	RESP	TEMP	Pulse O2	Glasgow Coma Scale Eye	Verb	Motor	Total	Revised Trauma Score (RTS) Resp	BP	GCS	Total	Revised Trauma Score Pediatric Resp	BP	GCS	Total
	/																
	/																
	/																
	/																

Respiratory Effort: ☐ 1 Normal ☐ 2 Shallow/Labored ☐ 3 Shallow/Non-Labored ☐ 4 Deep/Labored ☐ 5 Deep/Non-Labored ☐ 6 Absent ☐ 7 Labored/Fatigued ☐ **N Not Assessed** ☐ U Unknown

Resp. Sounds: L Clear R; L Bronchi R; L Rhales R; L Wheezes R

Skin Perfusion: ☐ 1 Normal ☐ 2 Decreased ☐ 3 **Not Assessed**

Pupils: L Normal R; L Constricted R; L Dilated R; L No react. R

Glasgow Coma Scale (GCS) Values

Eye Opening Component
0 Not applicable
1 None
2 Responds to Pain
3 Responds to Speech
4 Spontaneous Opening

Verbal Component
For patients >5 years:
1 None
2 Non-specific sounds
3 Inappropriate words
4 Confused conversation or speech
5 Oriented and appropriate speech
9 Unknown

For patients 2-5 years:
1 None
2 Grunts
3 Cries and/or screams
4 Inappropriate words
5 Appropriate words
9 Not assessed

For patients 0-23 months:
1 None
2 Persistent cry, grunting
3 Inappropriate cry
4 Cries, inconsolable
5 Smiles, coos, cries appropriately
9 Not assessed

Motor Component
For patients >5
1 None
2 Extensor posturing in response to painful stimulation
3 Flexor posturing in response to painful stimulation
4 General withdrawal in response to painful stimulation
5 Localization of painful stimulation
6 Obeys commands with appropriate motor response
9 Unknown

For patients up to 5 years
1 None
2 Extensor posturing in response to painful stimulation
3 Flexor posturing in response to painful stimulation
4 General withdrawal in response to painful stimulation
5 Localization of painful stimulation
6 Spontaneous
9 Not assessed

Revised Trauma Score (RTS) Values

Resp. Rate		Systolic B.P.		GCS Total	
10-29	4	BP>89	4	13-15	4
>29	3	76-89	3	9-12	3
6-9	2	50-75	2	6-8	2
1-5	1	1-49	1	4-5	1
None	0	None	0	< 4	0

Cardiac Arrest Information

Cardiac Arrest:	Y	N	**Bystander CPR:**	Y	N
Witnessed Arrest:	Y	N	**Pulse Restored:**	Y	N
Trauma Arrest:	Y	N	**Number of Shocks:**		

Cardio Pulmonary Arrest Time: ______

Min.	<4	<8	<12	>12	Unk.
Arrest to CPR:					
Arrest to DEFIB.					
Arrest to Meds.					

Cardiac Rhythm: I = Initial D = Destination PLEASE NOTE: ANY CHANGES IN CARDIAC RHYTHM SHOULD BE NOTED BELOW BY (↓ TIME COLUMNS)

I	D	↓ Time rhythm observed	I	D	↓ Time rhythm observed	I	D	↓ Time rhythm observed	I	D	↓ Time rhythm observed	I	D	↓ Time rhythm observed
		Not Applicable			AV Block - 1st			PEA (EMD)			PVCs			ST Elevation/Abnormal
		Unable to Identify			AV Block -2nd, Type I			Idioventricular			Sinus Bradycardia			SVT
		Asystole			AV Block -2nd, Type II			Junctional			Sinus Rhythm			Vent. Fibrillation
		Atrial Fibrillation			AV Block - 3rd			Pacemaker			Sinus Tachycardia			Vent. Tachycardia
														Other

Date: Signature ______

Typical Paramedic EMS form

Chapter Seven

Your primary diagnosis on a medical chart might well be whatever doctors get paid to call it

We operate under a well-known mantra when it comes to patient records: if we didn't write it down, it didn't happen. You can't get more basic than that.

The pre-hospital report is *the* tool for documentation of assessing and diagnosing, treating and dispensing care. Accurate charting is the justification for specific care, continued care and hopefully eventual payment. If it isn't recorded, it matters not at all whether the Paramedic performed, for example, an EKG on the side of the highway. We are going to need something that proves that we did what we said we did. The EMS record is simply the first of many pages known as "the chart."

Our vulnerable citizenry is under the illusion that patient medical charts are accurate and complete renditions of fact. After all, if we cannot trust health care, who can we trust?

Sadly, "wanting to believe" does not make it so. And there is yet a darker side to the inference noted above – namely, if we don't document it, we can pretend it didn't happen. Oh, there's more. By all measurable evidence, the most common 'fudging' going on is our third creative corollary: we can 'document' something happened even when it didn't happen at all. That proves that we were, you know, thorough.

One of medicine's shameful secrets is that patient charting information gets faked every day of the year, for any number of reasons. And some of the reasons can be pretty good ones. At least that is what we told ourselves when we were faking it. How often this happens is likely impossible to know. But over the past four years we've asked, and here is a small but representative peek at our question to a wide swath of medical professionals, followed by their responses:

"Are you aware of any medical staff fudging patient records for any reason at all?"

Their answers:

"The problem I see is medics short-cutting their own reports by using the automated E-narrative software. That often just does not describe their patient interaction in the least."
(NickelsMICN)

"When I'm in a hurry I use the vital signs that the nurses get before I leave as my final set on the patient. That way they always match and I can write that I did it twice."
(AMedic)

"I'm noticing now almost every time we get an ambulance report, the medic states the patient's respiratory rate is '20'. How can everybody have the same rate of breathing?"
(BessRN)

"I'm an EMT in a casino. It's an interesting place to work, to say the least. Very different from anything else I've done. I provide medical care, but my first duty is to protect the casino, like from crazy lawsuits. If an employee gets hurt, we start the worker's comp case, but we write it up to favor the casino, not the patient. So we're fudging all the time."
(Esse)

“I hate to say this out loud, but I work in LTC (note: long term care facility) and nurses are expected to be liars here. We generally have 40 patients each. There is no way in the world either the day shift or the PM shift can possibly do all that is required. We tell our RN supervisors all the time that we can only complete 40% of our work. They shrug and order us to initial each treatment item on the chart, as if it got done. At least our audits look good.”
(GreyCat)

“On our med-surg floor we've learned that honesty comes with consequences that will eventually get you fired. We work as hard as we can; fudge the rest; hoping for the best.”
(FYoungLVN)

“Falsifying documentation is serious business and nurses can lose their licenses over it. You can be sure if something goes wrong and the doo-doo hits the fan, the admins who told you to lie are not going to step forward and take the fall. I did it early in my career. I changed employers so I no longer have to do it. And I sleep a lot better these days.”
(Shelby)

“I've been asked by my superior to document lies concerning a resident's fall; that his V/S (vital signs) were within normal range; that he was not confused; that the bed rails were up; he sustained no injury, etc., etc. I was yelled at. 'We have a duty to protect this company!!!!' I refused to do it. The result for refusing? I was demoted, belittled and eventually fired 'at will.'”
(Letty)

“Everyone talks about the state coming and us getting in trouble for false documentation. I don't think the state cares because they have to know this goes on constantly all over this county.”
(JKE)

“The thing people have to understand it that EMS is so regulated – like a nuclear power plant. There is no possible way that medics – no matter how dedicated – can do all EMS regulates us to do, in the time we have with the patient. We spend so much

time 'proving' we did everything that there's no time do what we just documented we did. It's insane."
(BigBen)

"Evening in Milwaukee. The call is dispatched as 'nausea/vomiting with dizziness.' We arrive to find a male adult sitting in a car on the side of the road. He's been feeling this way for a couple hours and takes several cardiac medications. I find a blood pressure of 92/60. Way, way too low. Pulse is rapid, respirations are rapid and shallow. He's had an MI in the past. This man is seriously ill. As I'm assessing him, his implanted defibrillator begins to fire off, which means his heart has gone into a dangerous rhythm. We follow protocol and call Paramedics. This is a mixed blessing. On the one hand, ALS responders have a bigger bag of tools and great training. On the other hand, our fire department medics – plainly put – hate EMS. Paramedics here are, for the most part, firefighters who want to fight fires, not heart disease.

When they arrive we give our report, and the medic directs one of the firefighters to get a set of vitals. I stand by and watch. He turns around and tells the Paramedic, '120/80.' In Milwaukee, this is what we call, 'Engine 12ing the vitals.' Make 'em up out of thin air. Our ER docs and nurses use the phrase, too. It's a common phrase here because it's a common event. *Milwaukee fire medics make up the vital signs on patients.*

I cannot imagine how these people get away with this year after year. It's falsifying patient reports. Unacceptable. It should be criminal. This is a cardiac case. The next step might well be to administer nitroglycerin, which is contraindicated in patients with a systolic pressure under 100. This guy is at 92, but the Paramedic has just been told it's 120. If the guy gets nitroglycerin, he might die. In the end, the medic used my 92/60 finding as a guide on how to treat the fellow. But he didn't like it at all."
(Todd D)

"For me, I shouldn't even work in the clinic I'm at now, but I sure do love working with the elderly. Here, when a nurse leaves a blank space on a treatment that did not get done, the

medical records staff just forge the nurses' initials to make the chart appear complete."
(Anson)

"Falsify a PCR? Nah, I can't do it. I've been hassled to do it a few times by supervisors. I just tell them if they want science fiction they can write it themselves. I'll probably find out someday my PCRs have been totally rewritten."
(BarryPara)

"My advice to patients: when you check your medical records, do you see anything that doesn't jibe? Times, doctor's orders, procedures, signature page. Every order and comment needs to be validated throughout the chart. I had a case where one of my nurses went a week after a patient died in the ER and inserted charting notes to cover everyone's butt. The way we discovered it was that she messed up by automatically putting the current date on the notation."
(LaraBSN)

"Crews at our busy ambulance company write a paper chart at the time of call. On return to the station, some charts are entered into emsCharts by office staff. When info goes into emsCharts by a third-party, that name shows on the record as a crew member. Management claims this is necessary because crews are 'too busy' to enter their own charts. An offsite billing company downloads the PCR from emsCharts for billing. The electronic chart is the basis for billing Medicare, Medicaid & insurances. A copy may be viewed in an audit or trial. But a printout gives the impression that three people were on the call, when in fact there were only two. Management claims this is simply transcription, like an MD dictation. I think this practice is asking for trouble."
(JimEMT)

"Some things are just plain hard to handle. I've been working in a SNF (note: skilled nursing facility) for four years. We have certain vitals that are supposed to be taken at exact times. We have 10 patients each. Those times can be impossible to meet when unexpected things come up with other patients. The

nurse orienting me in the beginning just said, 'Sometimes you have to lie a little.' So we make up vital signs on stable patients, so we have more time with the really sick ones."
(NurseBedlam)

"Yes. I personally was fired for not lying on an EMS form. We had a nasty head-on collision call where a doctor on-scene absolutely made a mess out of what should have been a fairly clean triage. My partner & I could have run that call with no problem. I wrote up exactly how he acted on-scene and what the negative patient consequences were. My supervisor was actually a decent woman and she was ordered to get rid of me. She told me if I went quietly and did not pursue an unfair termination, she would give me a 'good reference' at the next ambulance company I applied for. And she did. I never would have gotten the great position I have now without that reference. But the subject of fake medical charting needs to be aired, and I regret I'm too cowardly to risk my job over it."
(LewisnStLouis)

"We do the best we can, but we are dealing with human beings, and sometimes their needs don't meet our supervisor's day planner."
(JK)

"I've always suspected the higher up you go on the educational food chain, the less common it is. I've heard of it happening, but doubt much creative writing is going on in our ICU. These people are true pros."
(Annie)

"I've seen way too many EMTs who have no idea how to take a decent set of vital signs. And God help them if their electronic

B/P cuff fails. They couldn't hear a weak diastolic to save themselves, let alone a patient."

(Aidey)

"Once when I was too exhausted to even eat I accidentally picked up the wrong chart and wrote an entire narrative on the wrong patient. A week later I realized what I'd done and examined both charts side-by-side. They could not have been more different in histories, diagnoses or care. My bad entry should have set off alarm bells to any RN with a brain. Sadly, nobody even noticed."

(Dreamkeeper)

"I've had any number of strange experiences. I once did follow-up vital signs about three minutes after a CNA documented a B/P of 120/80. The real blood pressure was 196/108. That's criminal. Did management do anything? Nope. The CNIs still walking the halls here, still taking vital signs on really sick people who deserve better."

(CVMurseNary)

"There is no point in falsifying vitals and I don't know anybody who does it. Of course I work in an ER. I think we're pretty damned ethical."

(KayRN)

"Our hospital stopped allowing CNAs to do glucose sticks because – are you ready for this – they were faking BLOOD SUGAR levels!!! Jeezus H. Christ."

(Lucky2BHere)

"I've seen fake info on charts before, yes. Some people have no class."

(RNMom)

"I always get the fastest set of vitals on patients coming through the door by Paramedics, because frankly I can't trust them like I used to. Where in the heck did quality EMS go, anyway?"

(PamMICN)

"One of my biggest peeves is blood pressures and sometimes you really can't get one. We use the electronic reports and they won't let us submit the report at all unless you have two sets of vitals for the patient. I don't like it but I understand why people fudge a B/P when they have no choice."

(NuBoy)

"This all sounds like BIG trouble. Charting is one of the most hated functions in EMS. I hate it too, but it is a necessary evil. I do often have my EMT partner enter demographics and other basic info for my charts on busy days. But I always check for accuracy."

(AgMedic)

"Lots of stuff gets fudged here. I doubt it's the facility's fault because it's really one of the nicest ones around and we've got great managers. We do it because it's easier than patient care. Most of us are pretty lazy."

(JessT)

"I once had a brief job in a facility where the aides would chart the same weight as last time on any difficult patient. I was an aide then and was told this is how it is done. I told a nurse manager about it before I left. I hope something was done. Just saying, sometimes there are people who think that this is ok to do. I've seen RNs chart clear lungs on patients who NEVER have clear lungs and no edema on people who ALWAYS have it. Sheesh. Some people don't even look. They chart like facts are not important."

(Carrie)

"From now on I'll get my own vitals on patients coming in the door via the medics. I did not realize that fudging vitals was so prevalent. I'm horrified."

(TummyTuck)

"I have run into this problem many times with vitals being faked, especially on a patient with issues, like high or low B/P, irregular heart rate, etc. Heaven forbid you should have to call a doc more than once in a night shift. That scares nurses silly."

(SugarComa)

"I watched a CNA pushing the Dinamap in and out of rooms. When I asked her for vitals on a patient, since they were not on the chart, she made a show of looking at her paper and when she couldn't find it she proceeded to tell me that she would just make up numbers. That statement sent cold shivers down my spine! Oh, she's still working. I was told good staff is hard to come by. No wonder health care is such a mess."

(Duchess)

"I moved to O.R. years ago to get as far as I could from this kind of nonsense. And I can promise you – at least in our house – that garbage behavior wouldn't last a full shift."

(AndynScrubs)

"I had admissions actually discharge my patient as 'dead' once. I understand how anybody can make a mistake. What I couldn't get was why they felt the need to argue with me, when I told them I was feeding the patient lunch as we talked."

(Pepper)

"I was visiting my mother at a rest home when she suddenly became dizzy for no apparent reason, so they called 911. When the medics arrived they could not get the automatic B/P cuff to work. They went and got another one and still no success. There happened to be a cuff on a table so I suggested they take her pressure manually. They looked at me like they honestly did not understand. I thought . . . don't people know how to take B/Ps by hand anymore? Are we all on autopilot these days?"

(MarianRetiredRN)

"I went into a room and found a patient near death, with her respirations no more than five per minute. A CNA had just left the room after charting the poor women's breathing rate as '18-20.' I was fuming when I took it to the nurse manager, but nothing was ever done."

(Zippy)

"I'm a LVN on a pediatric floor. I'm guessing it doesn't happen here, although two years ago they fired an LVN faking chart info on a medical floor."

(Bennie08)

"CNAs have been making up vital signs around this place as long as I've been here. I can remember once when all 28 patients

in our unit were breathing at exactly 20 breaths per minute. What are the cosmic odds of THAT?"
(Jennie)

"I can promise you that any facility that doesn't have an assertive risk manager, has sloppy charting going on and probably worse."
(NurseTim)

"When my wife had back surgery she worked at an Anonymous Ethics hotline at a trauma center for a year, fielding calls and inputting them for follow-up. The horror stories she'd relate when she'd get home every day shocked even me. And I'm a homicide investigator."
(RobRoy)

"I am soooo glad all my kiddoes are on monitors that interface with computer charting. Relying on people who could fake vital signs when they're busy is something I will never go back to. Yikes!"
(Dreamer)

"Two points to contribute: I'm rounding and approach a corner in the hall. I stop because I can hear the following: CNI1: 'I can't get a blood pressure on that patient. What should I do?' CNI2: 'Just write 120/80. That's always a good number.'

And that's exactly what I found on the patient record. So for those tepid souls who think medical charts are squeaky clean? Trust me: this is probably one of the very best hospitals in America, all and all, but our staff write more fiction than Stephen King."
(GreenTea)

"The other day I was taking care of a patient who was brought into the ER following a car crash. She was in spinal precautions and complained of neck and leg pain. Our ER physician arrived and did his exam from the doorway, holding his Tablet PC, checking off items into the Electronic T-sheet while he asked a few basic questions. He was in and out in less than a minute.

Later, out of curiosity, I reviewed the chart. Not surprisingly there was a comprehensive assessment: abdominal findings, lungs sounds, heart sounds, pupils and ocular movements,

neuro exam – all beautifully documented, all normal. Not bad for an exam conducted from the doorway. 100% bullshit. I watched without comment throughout the day and noticed the same general 'virtual' exam pattern on most of his patients and the same comprehensive documentation. About half the docs in our ER operate in a similar way although he is the worst. Others actually go so far as to perform the exams."
(EDMurse)

❖

We are gratified by the number of doctors generous enough with their time to weigh in on this subject. Their observations and experiences are truly invaluable to any serious critique of medicine's status quo. Some of their narratives were longer than we would have preferred, but we had no desire to take what they said out of context, so here you have it, word for word:

"In most areas of medicine you encounter fairly mundane diagnoses. A primary care physician might see 30 patients per day – 25 of whom come in for cholesterol, blood pressure or sugar checks. In psychiatry however, each day brings with it a chance to meet the nation's greatest citizens. Just this past week I met the inventor of the Knight Rider car, three millionaires, and a four-star general in the Air Force, who assured me that his commitment to the hospital was a mistake and that everything would be okay if I would just contact the Pentagon.

While documentation is important in any field, I've learned the art of 'buffing a chart' on this rotation. On every other rotation we students diligently note all of the patient's complaints, disease history and findings on exam. We do not bend any of the patient's information, nor do we editorialize to make the patients seem sicker than they are. On Psych rotation we try to make the patients seem as ill as possible. 'Buffing' is adding information that was not stated by the patient; not found on exam, or is simply untrue, for the sole purpose of trying to sway the reader in a particular direction. An example in the ER might be a patient who comes in with shortness of breath. To get the person examined by a cardiologist, you might

also say that the patient has chest pain once an abnormal EKG is discovered. Buffing is highly illegal but is practiced by many physicians to varying extremes."
(Anonymous)

"I hate doing it, but at times there is simply no option."
(R. Romanek)

"I recently started my career at one of the most prestigious clinics in the nation. I'm not seeing any need whatsoever to 'buff the charts' and frankly hope I never do."
(RadRufus)

"I can't even count how many times I've witnessed RNs, LVNs, and CNAs just scribble down an imaginary vital sign and walk out of the room. I've reached the point where I don't even care. I just do it over, to satisfy myself that what I notate is a correct rendition of fact."
(RonnieResident)

"I can assure you that we physicians love EMRs (electronic medical records) templates because they make documentation faster and easier. But abuses, such as cloning and 'exploding' notes, are taking us all down a very bad road in health care. If too much information is replicated from one EMR to the next, there is little to distinguish patient encounters, and that undermines physician attempts to establish medical necessity – the foundation of Medicare reimbursement – and definitely degrades quality of care."
(1ConcernedDoc)

"Well you gotta give us doctors a little room to fudge! It's apparent to me that in general, professionals resist when controls are so strict we can't do our jobs. Having a little deviation is acceptable. To err is human, right? We can't totally alleviate the tension that politics put on healthcare. Yet, there is a responsibility for those in healthcare to be better.

Fudging on a stable patient can give you more time to spend on those who aren't. Others will argue this, but there is such a thing as good fudge, used judicially."
(SamIamMD)

"I never, ever, ever fudge on a medical record. That would be immoral. I have been known to repair, overhaul, refurbish, botch, tinker and add a bit more detail later. Thank you for allowing me the opportunity to clarify."
(Teresi)

"I do Q5 calls and work 16 hours a day even when I'm off. My time sheet says I work 8:30 a.m. to 4:30 p.m. five days a week. In the beginning I filled out my time sheet honestly and was ordered to redo it. I was told in the real world it doesn't work that way. We are ordered to record the hours we are supposed to work, not the hours we actually work. Welcome to the world of residency."
(Psymed)

"I am on my way to averaging waaaay over 80 hours a week this rotation. When I brought this to the attention of my chief, it was implied we are expected to fake the numbers."
(Weeble)

"You've got to hand it to us – we absolutely love to intimidate. One way we do this is by speaking and writing in clichés and then nodding in agreement to our educated profundity. Patients are too scared to ask questions. I love it."
(BeachMD)

"I'm all for playing by the rules and someday, when I have my own practice, I plan to do just that. But I can promise you this: try pulling a 'whistleblower' routine in a trauma center and your next job will be family practice in Gwigillingok, Alaska."
(NidelQ)

"When I was young and naïve I used to wonder why all the residents at a big teaching facility didn't just walk en mass to a news conference on the sidewalk and tell the world exactly what is going on. I learned why when I got here. Specialties are very closed communities and you will be going back to your program for references and fellowships for years to come. That isn't a bridge you're willing to burn. You can do far more good once you're out on your own. First you have to get there."
(SchmorlsNode)

"There is always fear of retribution if you rock the boat among colleagues. Every time an MD applies to a hospital for privileges, the little matter of, 'is he or she a team player?' invariably comes up. Medicine is a lot like the Stockholm Syndrome, actually."
(L2D2)

"The matter of learning early on how to 'fudge' will only be fixed by junior-level whistleblowers willing to martyr themselves for the cause."
(EricTheRed)

"I'm in grad school getting my PhD in Social Work. I currently intern in a program at a *Veterans* location. I find that I'm constantly, uh, how to say this, polishing, my notes. Instead of documenting that someone is having 'aggressive' thoughts, for example, I sometimes use the term 'homicidal.' When they need to be hospitalized, I sprinkle the word 'homicide' in the notes. Some people should not be out walking around and creative writing is the only thing that keeps them out of Walmart with a knife on a Sunday night."
(Gleason)

"My chief makes it very clear that we are to chart our findings and log our hours honestly. I am grateful to be in a program that is so responsive to resident needs."
(Impromptu)

"I am stunned at how many training programs have people lie about their hours worked. Actually encouraging med students to start lying while they're in school? These trash bins need to be shut down!"
(Maceo)

"I doubt we will ever be caught because the laws protecting mental health charts are different than those for medical charts. In regular medicine, a patient has access to all of the information in his chart. Mental health notes, on the other hand, cannot be revealed to a patient due to the sensitive nature of what they contain. Therefore, we already have one of layer protection separating our 'buffed' notes from the patient's inquisitive eyes.

Further, if a court orders us to turn over our notes, a patient is going to have a hard time arguing that he does not suffer from 'persecutory delusional disorder.' We've done such an amazing job painting our patients as psychotic, antisocial murderers that I'm sure we could charge admission fees for lectures on how to 'buff a chart.' We could qualify anybody to be a psych patient here."
(Danno)

"Have never been in a situation where I was so rushed I couldn't keep it real. I'm sure it happens, though. More likely in the hectic inner-city facilities where they get bombed daily by floods of humanity."
(TKimmie)

"Speaking from inside the military system, I can tell you it is actually far easier to complain within the walls, and not go outside. They take fictitious records very seriously, and will listen when you speak out. Go Army!"
(Gastrapathy)

"Trust me: You learn early that if you get a reputation as a whiner, medicine has a very long memory. So write what you're told to write."
(BluAlien)

"I don't fake anything and I don't tolerate anyone around me who might do so. It all starts and ends at the top."
(ClarkKentMD)

"I write no science fiction, ever. But to be fair, in residency I did what I had to do and charted the way they wanted me to. And that included ten tons of crap. Some MDs fake it now because they did so much of it in training. My experience was just the opposite: it affected me so strongly that I vowed I would never fake the charts on my own patients the way we did in school."
(ProudnKansas)

❖

Otherwise ethical people doing highly unethical things. In medical charting this habit is baseline normal, yet far too many of my colleagues keep sipping the wicked soup of denial. I understand completely. I sipped it myself for a long, long time.

❖

Convictions piling up for OrthoFix bone growth corporation

In May 2013, the *U.S. Attorney's Office* in Massachusetts announced that Hunter Rigsby, a former manager, admitted to health care fraud and paying kickbacks to doctors during a six-year period beginning in 2005. Rigsby sold Orthofix bone growth stimulators in Tennessee.

According to the court record, Medicare reimburses for "long bone" stimulators only after 90 days have elapsed without clinically significant healing, and only covers certain types of injuries. Rigsby was well aware of these guidelines. But he sold doctors bone growth stimulators that did not satisfy Medicare's guidelines.

The *U.S. Attorney's* office said some physicians would prescribe the device before 90 days had elapsed without any healing; others for patients who had injuries that were not covered under Medicare's guidelines. When this occurred, *Rigsby would forge the patient's medical records* to make it appear as though the claim was payable under Medicare's guidelines.

Rigsby admitted in court he also deleted portions of patient chart notes describing injuries not covered by Medicare. He also forged physicians' signatures on prescriptions and Medicare Certificates of Medical Necessity.

Prosecutors said Rigsby's scam caused Medicare and other insurance programs to pay more than $400,000 for bone growth stimulators that should not have been paid.

❖

"In psychiatry 'buffing' is a perfectly acceptable part of medicine. On any given morning I might round on a patient who tells me that he no longer hears voices and has no thoughts of hurting himself or others. He might say he wishes to be discharged so that he can go home and live his life. The nurse's report might state the patient has been perfectly cooperative; that he has

mostly kept to himself; that he slept throughout the night without any intervention or extra medication. But in his chart I will state that the patient continues to respond to internal stimuli; (note: he's hearing voices) that he is isolated and withdrawn; and that he needs continuous 24-hour monitoring to ensure that he is not a danger to himself or others. This practice of "buffing the charts" is not only encouraged – it's required – by my superiors. It's just the way it is."
(PsyPhi)

"'If it isn't charted, it isn't done,'" is simply an impossible rule to satisfy. Since what could be charted is infinite, I begin each shift knowing that I have already failed in my documentation. I make up for it by astuteness. Next."
(Internalizer)

"I had this exact conversation about fictitious charting with my nurse-wife the other day. I argued there is no way the average person takes a breath every three seconds. At the *VA* when I was in training, every person had an R/R of '20' no matter what. It was expected, and it was science fiction."
(HappyHospitalist)

❖

Louisiana physician confesses to 35 counts of Medicaid fraud

In the city of Kenner a doctor has pleaded guilty to nearly three dozen charges of fraud, after operating a scam out of his medical office aimed at stealing from the state's *Medicaid* program.

Doctor Fiaz Afzal, age 49, who owned the *Claiborne Medical Corporation* in Kenner, was arrested in January, 2010. A grand jury investigation revealed that he was routinely submitting fraudulent claims to the *Medicaid* program regarding patient claims, for the purpose of gaining greater compensation.

"Dr. Afzal used his medical license to take advantage of the state's insurance program, and more reprehensibly, his own patients," said Louisiana Attorney General Buddy Caldwell.

During the course of the investigation, the *Medicaid Fraud Control Unit* learned that for a 15-month period starting in January, 2009, Afzal "knowingly falsified documents to support fraudulent billing." He also wrote fake diagnoses for patients, in order to justify billing for exams and treatments that never happened.

Afzal faces a sentence of 175 years in federal prison upon sentencing by Judicial District Court Judge Trudy White, at a date to be determined.

❖

New Jersey doctor pleads guilty in health insurance fraud scheme

In the city of Trenton Criminal Justice Director Gregory Paw told reporters that a Hudson County medical doctor has *pleaded guilty to falsifying medical records.*

According to Insurance Fraud Prosecutor Greta Brown, Farouk Al-Salihi, 72, a physician in Jersey City, pleaded guilty yesterday before Superior Court Judge Peter Vazquez to criminal fourth-degree falsifying records in order for a patient to submit phony health insurance claims.

❖

Chicago surgeon convicted of falsifying patient records

A Chicago-area surgeon has been found guilty of lying, *falsifying patients' medical charts* and submitting false claims for payment to Medicare.

Doctor John Natale, age 63, worked at *Northwest Community Hospital* in Arlington Heights. He specialized in repairing abdominal aortic aneurysms. His trial focused on six surgeries he performed in 2003 and 2004. Prosecutors proved that Natale falsified post-operative reports on at least two patients by describing the surgeries he performed as being more complex than they were, and writing detailed descriptions of surgical repairs that he never performed.

At trial, another surgeon testified that after one of Natale's patient's health deteriorated, he had to sort through the lies in

Natale's reports and that the false statements could have seriously affected patient outcome.

Natale was sentenced to a 10-month prison term and a $40,000 fine.

❖

New Jersey doctor changes his mind; confesses guilt

In an unexpected move, the Morrisville Pennsylvania physician accused in a false prescriptions scam voluntarily pleaded guilty in the midst of his criminal trial Wednesday morning.

Doctor William Kropinicki, age 59, announced his guilt of all five charges against him, including unlawfully dispensing of a controlled substance; *falsification of medical records*; falsification of prescriptions and obtaining narcotics by fraud.

Investigators learned in 2008 that the doctor would routinely write narcotic prescriptions for patients he had never examined or even met. He would then *create fake medical records* of the so-called "patients."

Kropinicki's open guilty plea was followed by him being handcuffed by police officers immediately and taken to jail. He was sentenced to seven years in prison.

❖

Tennessee nurse convicted in false patient treatment records case

In the small Scott County city of Abington a nurse has been found guilty of *making false entries into an elderly patient's medical records.*

Melissa A. Forester was convicted of one count of making 'false statements related to a health care matter,' according to the U.S. Attorney's office. At the time of her arrest, Ms. Forester was employed as a licensed practical nurse at the *Brian Center Rehabilitation* facility in Weber City, where she had worked from 2006-2011.

According to the court records, a patient identified as 'Resident 31' developed numerous pressure ulcers on the lower back.

Nurse Forester not only failed to provide adequate care, but indicated on medical charts that the ulcerations were not serious.

Investigators learned otherwise when the patient was transported to a local emergency room, the physician found her wound dressing "full of feces" and severely infected. The patient died later at another nursing home.

In the indictment, prosecutors showed that Forester made entries in the patient's chart indicating she was administering regular treatment, including wound care, on days when she was not even present at the *Brian Center.*

❖

Paramedic and EMT admit participation in EMS recertification scam

In Boston Attorney General Martha Coakley has announced that a Paramedic and an EMT have been sentenced after pleading guilty for their roles in a training records scheme. They *falsely recorded* that dozens of EMTs attended mandatory continuing education classes to maintain their certification.

Victor Valdez, age 47 and Jeffrey Given, 42, confessed in Suffolk Superior Court their roles in the fraudulent EMT recertification scheme. EMT instructor Leo Nault, age 51, had already pled guilty to 16 separate charges of violations and conspiracy. Nault was given a 30-month suspended sentence and a $16,000 fine.

Valdez worked as an EMT and supervisor at *Armstrong Ambulance* in Arlington, Massachusetts. He collected signatures of Nault's attendance rosters from EMT coworkers, and obtained signatures of other public safety employees as well. He was sentenced to one year of probation on two counts of Conspiracy to Commit OEMS Violations. He was also ordered to pay $6,000 in fines.

Jeffery Given, from Haverhill, was a Paramedic at *Trinity Ambulance* and was also a firefighter. Given collected signatures from fellow firefighters on Nault's rosters. These refresher courses were either not taught, or were taught but not attended by the firefighters. Given was sentenced to a year of probation for Conspiracy to Commit OEMS Violations, and a $5,000 fine.

❖

Paramedics often take on second jobs and that has always been the case with me. The 24-hour 'Kelly' shift affords numerous benefits, not the least of which is 12-14 days off each month to pursue other interests. And I have dabbled in several. By far the most provocative was performing medical-legal casework for a company called *Great Western Medical Group* in Palm Springs.

Great Western specialized in workers' compensation medical examinations – patients who reported being injured on the job. Our 27 physicians in three offices performed what is called "defense" work, meaning we were hired by employers to determine if the employee injury complaints were legitimate and if so, how serious. As is typical in the business, our doctors were orthopedists for bone, muscle and ligament damage; neurologists for brain and nerve problems; ophthalmologists for eye trauma, and so on. They would assess incoming patients and dictate their findings. Transcribers would then type the reports and give them to us. As medical-legal editors we would proofread, copy-edit and – depending on the literacy of the physician – totally rewrite reports as necessary, to ensure each case was clear enough to meet the strict criteria of the courts. Simply put, the only reason our profession existed was because – as I learned soon enough – the typical workers' comp doctor appeared wholly incapable of dictating a record that could pass muster at the high school level.

Occasionally on Sunday mornings I found myself in my office when no one else was around, or so I thought. I discovered that happened to be when the psychiatrists slyly sneaked *their* patients in. Who knew? They would hold their sessions on the only day the rest of the clinic was closed; in the only office with a private back door – the office right next to mine. I soon realized that if I sat absolutely still, I could hear every word said between the psych docs and their patients. Some of the chats made me slosh my coffee.

As I worked my way up the ladder I was offered more and still more highly complex cases. But I never did reach the point of rewriting psychiatric evaluations, because they were the trickiest of the bunch. All of the psych editing at *Great Western* went to my mentor – a funny, acerbic fellow named Cary Lynch. Cary worked out of the main office in Riverside and we often played basketball on the court at Sonny Bono's restaurant. One day he dropped by to pick up his files. It was quite a stack, so I asked him about it. We all worked on tight deadlines and what he had in his hands looked to be a Herculean task.

He shrugged. "Fourteen files this time. I've had worse."

I said, "We have two psych-meisters here, right?"

"Yeah, but one of them's out for a while, so these are all from one guy."

"And they only come in on Sunday mornings."

"I didn't know that."

"Well, they do. I don't know what they look like because they come and go through their own back door."

"Sounds like a psych. They are different."

I shook my head, still staring at his pile of cases. I asked, "Mind if I take a look at a couple of these?"

Cary shrugged again. "Sure. HIPPA won't mind a bit."

I grinned and started thumbing slowly through a pair, then handed them back.

"You do realize, I'm sure, being my mentor and all, that those 15-18 page transcriptions are bullshit, right?"

"Of course. They're psych reports. Psych is the acme of medical bullshit. But how do *you* know they're bullshit?"

"Because the psych-meisters are never in there long enough to do 14 patients justice. I can hear every word of every exam. They don't dictate more than three sentences on anybody. They are in and out in two hours."

Cary looked down at his pile. "No wonder they're so easy to do. Those guys are telling the transcribers to use templates on the patients."

"Same templates? Same diagnoses?"

"Pretty much, yeah."

I shook my head. "How much do these clowns make per exam?"

"First time patient? Comprehensive work-up? $1492.00."

"Comprehensive?"

I glared out the window of the clinic at the pristine Palm Springs street known as Tahquitz Canyon. I thought I was doing a pretty fair job of staying under control, because I had an overwhelming desire to toss a chair through that very expensive glass, just to see if anybody would recognize crappy behavior when they saw it. I wasn't sure anybody would.

Instead, I spoke to my buddy through gritted teeth. "Cary, doesn't it piss you off even a little bit that these lab coat lunatics are ripping off the entire system to the tune of $10,000 an hour?"

❖

I wanted to leave it alone, I really did. But the outright gall of these freaky fraudsters was making me a little crazy. MDs unable explain the difference between a symptom and a diagnosis were getting rich playing the workers compensation *Bowling for Dollars* sport. Psychiatric quacksalvers – spending a whole three minutes with patients before playing God with their lives – were amassing wealth by churning out head game flummery. I did not yet know that I was edging toward the maelstrom of one of the biggest medical scams in California history. I did know I was a key player in garbage health care; that we were toying with the lives of thousands of patients and it needed to be stopped. But it did not take long to verify what I viscerally knew already – that *Great Western* management was not about to start clashing with physicians over the way they conducted their exams. When it came to company profit, challenging doctors was the fast-track to corporate suicide. As Cary Lynch advised me during a bruising game of one-on-one, there was gold in the mother lode of workers' compensation, and neither *Great Western*, nor any of the other case management heavy hitters, was about to rock the money boat.

It was about a month later, I think, before a plan of attack began to crystallize in my weary head. For weeks I'd taken to jotting down names of people I had known over the years, particularly those with some measure of clout in whatever circle they moved in. But I could not recall anyone with the interest or the power to meet this challenge head-on, let alone actually help clobber some bad guys. Sonny Bono was in Congress now although he was a possibility, somebody in California would be quicker.

Then one morning while driving across the desert to work, the answer hit me like a pie, smack in the face. I got so excited I actually pulled off the highway and took a few deep breaths. I stared at a sand dune. The man who had spearheaded the San Diego City Paramedic program years before was Mayor Pete Wilson. In the earliest stages, Wilson's city council was under serious pressure for women medics to be schooled, hired and trained. And that idea received more than a little resistance. Absolutely nobody wanted women in the city's 40 fire stations overnight, for one thing. As San Diego's first EMS field supervisor, I was asked personally by the mayor to take a temporary assignment – to mentor and partner the first female Paramedic in the city's history, in that first year. In order to keep the furor to a minimum, the city made an agreement to house this male/female team at *Mercy Hospital*. Like every other medic in the county, I wanted nothing to do with female partners. But when a man like Pete Wilson pulls up in a limousine and asks you for a professional favor, you usually do it. And as we shook hands, damned if he hadn't said this:

"Consider yourself a city patriot. And I'll owe you one."

Yes, indeed. And it just so happened that Peter Barton Wilson was now the sitting Governor of the State of California. And he owed me one.

Sometimes – not often – the idea of an interactive God seems plausible.

❖

And so it came to pass that by the end of that year Governor Pete Wilson and I met twice – once in Los Angeles; once in

Palm Springs – brief visits while he was on trips for other reasons. He remembered our meeting years before and we chatted about the early successes of San Diego's EMS system. I told him three of the first four lady medics turned out just fine. We talked about *PSA Flight #182* and how horrible it had been. He was gracious and quick to grasp the subject at hand. No need to remind him he owed me a favor; he would never have agreed to meet me at all, if he himself had not recalled our brief history. This time he introduced me to one of his assistants, who in turn asked me to provide any proof at all of my "suspicions." On the second visit I handed the assistant tape recordings of our psychiatrists' sham patient assessments, (complements of a Radio Shack listening device I'd attached to my office wall) as well as a large envelope full of copies of workers' comp medical reports, all of which I had totally rewritten, part and parcel to my job. Included were copies of the original physician transcriptions, gobbledygook and all, for comparison. The ladies in transcribing had been reluctant at first, but in the end, they too were weary of all the lying. The Governor and his aide agreed that no physician should be paid for sloppy reports, and the industry norm of total rewrites by editors had to be illegal on several levels. I had photographs of the psych-meisters' arrival on Sunday mornings and time-stamped their departures. Their scam was obvious too: no one can adequately workup 14 patients and then dictate full reports on each, in two hours. We shook hands all around. We agreed to stay quiet and stay in touch.

Although I had no way of knowing it, the Governor had already taken a keen interest in California workers' compensation fraud. They had a task force in place. What they were looking for was proof from the trenches, and by the Spring of the year they had more than they needed. The Governor was finally able to move on the reform he had wanted since entering office. He signed Senate Bill 31 that year, which placed severe limits on the fees paid to doctors and medical firms for medical-legal evaluations. His legislation created felony punishment for workers' compensation fraud and provided state funding to the *Department of Insurance Bureau of*

Fraudulent Claims. It also provided money to county district attorneys to investigate and prosecute scam doctors and "medical mills."

Clinics Raided in Massive Workers' Comp Probe:
Search Warrants Served at 150 California Sites
July 01, 1993 | STUART SILVERSTEIN and ERIC YOUNG | L.A. TIMES STAFF WRITERS

❖

The impact of what we – along with other unknown exasperated professionals behind the scenes – accomplished, became apparent almost immediately. The sordid subject was prime-time news fodder for weeks. The effect was particularly visible in Southern California, where 75 bustling clinics churning out mephitic medicine, were shut down. And by golly, our very own *Great Western Medical Group* was one of them.

"The fraud program is working very well. Although arrests have leveled off now, convictions are going up. We're very pleased about the way the fraud legislation is working."
Willie Washington, Director of Workers' compensation
State of California

"For years, California's fraud-ridden workers' compensation system has been the single greatest barrier to job creation in this state. But today, we're starting the process of tearing down that barrier, freeing Californians to create tens of thousands of new jobs a year."
Governor Pete Wilson
Sacramento press conference

❖

So the gratifying result was that we nailed just about a thousand arrogant turds and stopped at least one daffy doc gravy train in its tracks. Some of them – not nearly enough – took short detours to state prison, including one of our very own Sunday morning psychiatrists. Sorry to interrupt your golf game, doc. The entire adventure makes me smile, even two decades later. The nifty listening device sits in a drawer as I write this, comfortably retired. I should spray the thing gold and frame it. Of course the bad news was I very effectively worked my way right out of a terrific second income, and how smart is that, really? Regardless, Sonny Bono's words were never more appropriate:

"Sometimes you've just got to out-sneak the bastards."

❖

And finally, we say this. For any experienced health professional to even utter a doubt that this subject is pervasive, is to feign a level of naiveté that simply does not exist in the world of medicine. False documentation strikes at the heart of all the good we do. It is real and it is ubiquitous. No health care organization would condone tinkering with patient records out loud and they ought not tolerate the practice behind closed doors. But they do. They do it by sending mixed signals to staff who cannot possibly reconcile time versus accuracy. They do it because they have learned the hard way that cheating protects them from oversight agencies at audit time. They do it because lots of times they have simply not hired staff with the scruples it takes to function honestly every hour of every day.

The patient care industry is not even close to the transparency needed to change this disgrace. And transparency is the only way it will ever right itself. To date there is precious little collective effort to be more responsive to patients and families, for example, when disputes arise over the veracity of charting. All of this needs to change, but we are not even slightly hopeful it will occur anytime soon. Like alcoholism, you first admit you have a problem. And there exists no more denial of truth in health care than this:

Immutable Law #7

Should you count on your medical chart being 100% true? Absolutely not. There's more fiction in health care than Barnes & Noble at Christmastime.

"I want to sell drugs to everybody. I want to sell drugs to healthy people. I want drugs to sell like chewing gum."

—Henry Gadsden
Former Chief Executive Officer
Merck Pharmaceuticals

Chapter Eight

We call it 'pharmageddon.' And damned few patients have a clue the real reason they are taking their pills, is because some drug rep happened to have seriously world-class legs.

Listen to me. You don't work in this business for long before you notice the sexy parade of sales reps breezing through doctor waiting room doors. Neither must you be Sherlock Holmes to deduce that if the physician is male, the rep will be female, and unfailingly striking. And vice versa. I'm here to report that the impact of suntanned legs waltzing through Palm Springs clinics can honestly make you short of breath.

While researching another subject a few years ago, we stumbled upon a curious aspect of pharmaceutical gamesmanship in America. It turns out that a curious number of drug reps are former college cheerleaders. Imagine that. According to author Jamie Reidy, women in drug sales have a clear advantage over their male counterparts, when it comes to breaking down objections by physicians. And Reidy would probably know. He was a successful salesman himself with

Pfizer, until he was terminated after writing a rather scathing book on the drug industry, entitled *Hard Sell: The Evolution of a Viagra Salesman.*

In an interview Jamie Reidy recalled a sales visit when he once accompanied the "all-time most attractive, coolest woman in the history of drug repdom." At first, he said, it looked like the sale was just not going to happen. "The doctor came up with about 10 reasons not to use one of our drugs." But eventually, Reidy added, "my partner gave a little hair toss and a tug on his arm and said, 'Come on, doctor, I need the sale.'

That MD completely gave in to this gorgeous woman, saying, 'Okay, how do I dose this drug?'

There is absolutely no way I could ever reach out and touch a female physician that way."

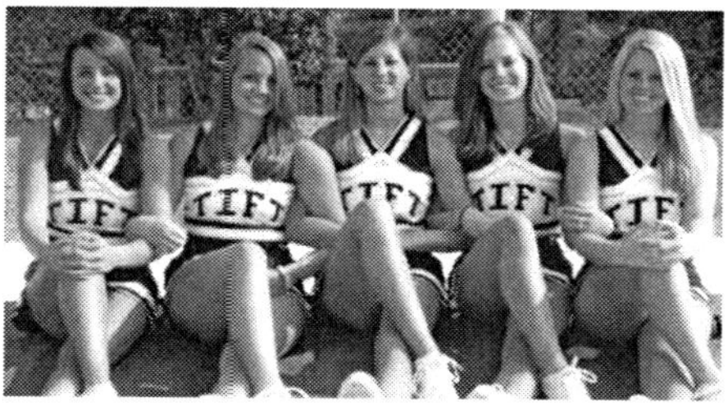

Tell us again why you think you're taking those pills (Photo Credit: Mark Larson studios)

Cheerleaders. And now they are going pro in more ways than one. They pep up the crowds for the Jets and the Chargers and the Lakers and the Dolphins on Sunday afternoons. They pep up doctors on Monday mornings. No need to take our word for it. Check out the website of a company calling itself *Spirited Sales.* Why, the whole idea just makes us want to stand up and cheer.

You Are Hired!

Congratulations to these *Spirited Sales* candidates on their success in landing new sales positions this year:

Novartis hired: Jennifer, Brandy, Charles, Angela, Brandi, Chelley, Emily, Lindsey, Kristen, Jackie, Mindy and Shermin.

Sciele hired: Elizabeth, Darcy, Sarah, Laura, Kristy, Christina, Jenn, Alisha and David

Daiichi Sankyo hired: Ashley, Caitlin and Egle

Boeringer Ingleheim hired: Susannah, Kris and Katherine

ADP hired: Stephanie and Monica
Bayer hired: Kimberly and Alyana
Santaurus hired: Rebecca and Michelle
Leitner hired: Wendy, Kristi and Kenny
Innovex hired: Rob, and,
Mission Pharmacal hired: Alex
Way to go, cheerleaders! We're so proud of you!

❖

"There's a saying in medicine," says Doctor Thomas Carli of the *University of Michigan.* "You'll never meet an ugly drug rep."

Doctor Carli has led efforts to limit access to the short-skirted saleswomen who troll the corridors of his hospital. He went on record years ago, saying that seduction is a deliberate industry marketing strategy.

So what kind of an education best prepares you for a lucrative career in prescription drug sales?

"Nobody asks what their major is," says T. Lynn Williamson, a cheer adviser at the *University of Kentucky.* He says he regularly gets calls from recruiters looking for talent, mainly from pharmaceutical companies. "They watch to see who's graduating," he notes. "Proven cheerleading skills suffice. Exaggerated motions, exaggerated smiles, exaggerated enthusiasm. With those skills they can get doctors to do whatever they want."

❖

It is indeed a wicked symbiosis, this unholy marriage between MDs and the drug industry. But we in EMS pretend the cloaking is 'health care' and fake the reality. Paramedics do not choose the drugs and we don't prescribe them. We just push them every chance we get, and perform CPR on those whose pills for some reason just did not, you know, work too well.

❖

By the numbers

- How much did the drug industry spend on marketing directly to doctors last year? $1,000,000,000 a month. That's with a "B."

- Marketing versus research & development budget? 2 to 1
- Ratio of drug reps to doctors in North America: 1 to 2
- How often they say a drug rep can get doctors to use their drug as opposed to their competitors' after a three-minute visit? 52%

Sound like harmless, free-market fun and games? Only to the witless:

- We now have 2,000,000 prescription drug addicts in the U.S. We have 30 drug-addicted babies born every day
- When pregnant mothers get high, so do their babies, who then get agitated until they get their next drug fix
- Addicted mothers are actually told by their MDs to keep taking the drugs throughout their pregnancy so the babies don't go into withdrawals and die in the womb
- According to *DEA* Agent Tom Lenox in San Diego, "legal" prescription death rate is higher than alcohol, crack cocaine and heroin combined – 38,000 a year
- Hundreds of thousands of adults have been injecting oxycodone since they were teenagers
- Because pharmaceuticals are made in clean laboratories, addicts know they are "safer" in quality and content
- Snorting or injecting prescription narcotics creates the high. It also rewires the brain and guarantees addiction
- "Oxy," Percocet, Xanex, Vicoden, Tramadol – any drug the U.S. makes – can be bought cheaper south of the border, which creates an almost unfathomable financial engine
- 80 milligram "oxy" pills – Oxycodone – are the most popular and cost $35 per tablet – half the price as in the U.S
- One pill crushed and injected can kill a user

❖

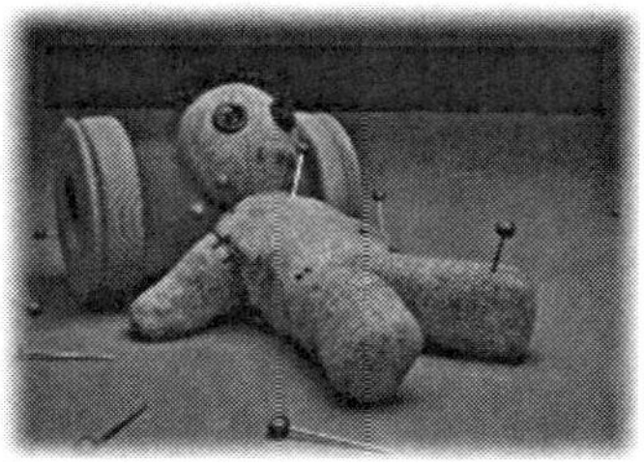

It's the drugs, dummy

Maybe you haven't noticed, but celebrities with more money than self discipline have been dropping like flies over the years. CPR didn't work on them, either. Here are but a few who allowed "health care" to lure them into early holes in a lawn:

Corey Haim, 38, actor
Brittany Murphy, 32, actress
Lesley Carter, 25, actress
Paul DeMayo, 37, bodybuilder
Eric Douglas, 36, actor, comedian
Gidget Gein, 39, musician
Peaches Geldof, 25, fashion model
Lisa Robin Kelly, 43, actress
Bobby Hatfield, 63, Righteous Brothers vocalist
Heath Ledger, 28, actor
John Pinette, 50, actor
Anna Nicole Smith, 39, former Playmate of the Year
Michael Jackson, 50, singer
Amy Winehouse, 27, musician
Steve Bechler, 23, Baltimore Orioles pitcher
Vic Chesnutt, 45, musician
Greg Geraldo, 44, comedian
James "Ultimate Warrior" Hellwig, 54, professional wrestler
Corey Monteith, 31, actor
Amy Tryon, 42, Olympic equestrian
Brian Adams, 38, singer/songwriter
Bridgette Andersen, 22, actress
Matthew Ansara, 35, actor, bodybuilder
Erica Blasberg, 28, professional golfer
John Belushi, 36, comedian
Len Bias, 23, basketball player
Elisa Bridges, 28, Playboy Playmate
Ken Caminiti, 42, baseball player
Andy Irons, 32, professional surfer
Christopher Bowman, 40, figure skater
Lisa Robin Kelly, 43, actress
Brian Epstein, 34, entertainment manager
Chris Farley, 33, comedian
Thomas Kincade, 54, artist
Adrienne Nicole Martin, 27, model
Danny Gans, 52, Las Vegas magician

Margaux Hemingway, 42, model
Mitch Hedberg, 37, comedian
Anissa Jones, 18, child actress
Chris Kelly, 34, musician
Derek Boogaard, 28, professional ice hockey player
Billy Mays, 51, TV salesperson
Michael Carl Baze, 24, horse jockey
River Phoenix, 23, actor
Dana Plato, 34, actress
Freddie Prinze, 22, actor, comedian
Rachel Roberts, 36, actress
Whitney Houston, 48, singer
Phillip Seymour Hoffman, 46, actor

❖

Across our southern border pharmacists and doctors in Tijuana are so used to seeing gringos walk through the doors asking for drugs that they don't even blink anymore. But these days they can offer something even better than illicit drugs, and something a street dealer cannot offer: long-term "legal" prescriptions, which can be used anywhere at any time. They are gifts that keep on giving.

In America the prescription drug epidemic is so out of control that addicts have no real reason to go as far as Mexico and risk a border search. Countless thousands of rogue doctors feed the need and every "patient" is a 24-hour ATM machine.

Would physicians actually risk losing their family, their kids, their careers, their respect? Oh, they do it every day. In 2002 Doctor James Graves of Florida became the first MD in history to be convicted of manslaughter in connection with the Oxycontin death of a patient. He was sentenced for the deaths of four patients who died from overdoses. Since then, more than 400 other physicians have also been convicted on various levels of drug pushing. Doctor/Drug-dealer. Our new, 21st Century American career path.

In the state of Florida alone, 40,000 MDs prescribe 80% of all pain pills in the nation. These "pill mills" fuel the epidemic.

Hundreds of big-time drug dealers have abandoned the illegal rackets of the past to get into the "legitimate" pill business with corrupt physicians. They know what doctors know: "pain" does not show up on an x-ray or an MRI. It does not reveal itself on a CT scan or a blood or urine test. So if a corrupt MD is even reasonably careful, he or she can sell drugs with impunity. By performing recordable exams, criminal physicians effectively cover their tracks and their behinds.

The feds do what they can. Jeanette Moran is a *Drug Enforcement* Agent in Florida who investigates criminal doctors. She tells us many of the clinic owners are former street drug pushers and have no problem hiring corrupt MDs with legal prescription pads. In a single *DEA* sweep called Operation Pill Nation in 2011, Moran and her colleagues arrested a dozen doctors operating five clinics that were bringing in a jaw-dropping $150,000 a day.

Because of the explosive growth of physician-generated drug-pushing, many states now have prescription drug tracking programs. Other states don't bother. But there is a strong reason for every state to have a Prescription Drug Monitoring Program. Nationwide, communities are being ripped apart by prescription drugs and EMS expends enormous resources responding to the human fallout. Adams County Ohio, for example, where this author was raised, has been devastated by drug abuse. Jails once rarely occupied by more than two or three arrestees, generally for small time offenses, are now full of drug addicts convicted of crimes to support their habits. Rural Adams County, with a population of less than 30,000, has the highest rate of prescription deaths in a state with such cities as Cleveland and Cincinnati, with 10 times the population.

Shamefully, thousands of unscrupulous doctors have amassed untold wealth as the direct result of the $320,000,000,000 prescription drug industry. And who gets the call on the 38,000 fatal drug overdoses each year? Paramedics. And I can promise you people are crying when we get there.

❖

Yes indeed, we Americans have a rapacious appetite for pills. We are the globe's greatest gobblers of psychotropic drugs, for one. We pop 6 out of every 10 on earth. That's 40,000,000 pills a day. Curious, isn't it? Every few weeks a madman pulls out an assault rifle and slaughters complete strangers. And we wonder why.

❖

Television network news chose to pretend it didn't happen, back in the Fall of 2009, for reasons known only to themselves. It was all but ignored in the print media, too – coast to coast, from the *Los Angeles Times* to the *Washington Post*. We recall our own exasperation at the time, but we were not surprised. The largest criminal fine in history had just been meted out to the largest drug maker on the planet. Pfizer would pay $2,300,000,000 as the result of criminal charges related to Bextra, an anti-inflammatory drug designed primarily for arthritis. The *FDA* had already forced Pfizer to stop selling the drug because of mounting evidence that it compounded the risk of brain damage, heart damage and death. And now Justice Department prosecutors had proven that Bextra, among other drugs, was marketed as treatment for medical conditions beyond its scope.

To those of normal sensibilities, the fact that Pfizer could possibly still be allowed – in the year 2014 – to sit at the table and poop in their adult pants, is perplexing. This was the fourth colossal scam they had been caught pulling in 10 years. Like the other three, the fine would amount to little more than a traffic ticket to a cartel that pilfers the public to the tune of $1,000,000,000 a week. The fine – as hefty as it sounds – was little more than a slap on the sassy butt. They turned around and bought Wyeth for $68,000,000,000 within three months.

In the upside down world of legal drug-running Pfizer may be the orca in the pool, but there are plenty of other predators in the water:

Cartels behaving badly

Bristol Myers Squibb
Fine: $500,000,000
Year: 2007
Drug involved: *Abilify*, an antipsychotic and Serzone, an anti-depressant
Criminal charges filed? No

BMS heavily marketed its antipsychotic Abilify to treat dementia in the elderly and to treat behavioral problems in children – conditions the drug was not approved to address. Also, despite a *Food and Drug Administration* warning about potentially fatal side effects of Abilify in the elderly, *BMS* sent sales teams to nursing homes to promote the drug anyway, and paid doctors to dispense them, enticing the unscrupulous with expensive vacations to luxury resorts. Why that isn't considered criminal is beyond our comprehension.

AstraZeneca
Fine: $520,000,000
Year: 2010
Drug involved: Seroquel, an antipsychotic
Criminal charges filed? No

AstraZeneca was charged with illegally marketing Seroquel to the elderly and to children; to treat conditions for which it had not been found safe, including insomnia and anxiety. AstraZeneca also promoted Seroquel for weight loss, while hiding data that showed that to the contrary, it caused weight gain – an average of nearly a pound a month. Other studies had repeatedly shown that Seroquel caused metabolic problems like diabetes. They got their hands slapped, but no one was seriously punished.

Purdue Pharmaceutical
Fine: $630,000,000
Year: 2007

Drug involved: *Oxycontin*, a painkiller
Criminal charges filed? Yes

Oxycontin was marketed as a pain relief narcotic in 1995, by Purdue Pharma, who made exaggerated claims that it was less addictive and less likely to cause withdrawals, than other similar medications. Purdue was charged with using misleading sales tactics, minimizing the risks of the drug and promoting it to treat types of pain for which it had not been appropriately studied. Bless their hearts.

Amgen
Fine: $762,000,000
Year: 2012
Drugs involved: *Aranesp* and *Epogen* for anemia
Criminal charges filed? Yes

Amgen was discovered to be deliberately overfilling Aranesp containers so that doctors could give the 'free' drugs to patients and then bill insurance companies for it. The company was also suspected of using the profits to bribe doctors to write prescriptions for Aranesp instead of for competing drugs. You just have to admire how creative these folks can get into other peoples' wallets.

Merck
Fine: $950,000,000
Year: 2011
Drug involved: The painkiller *Vioxx* (rofecoxib)
Criminal charges filed? Yes

Merck's Vioxx was ordered off the shelves in 2004 after research proved it doubled the risk of heart and brain damage. The company made false claims about the drug's safety and illegally promoted it for medical problems for which it had not been properly tested, such as rheumatoid arthritis. A federal investigation revealed Vioxx contributed to approximately 50,000 deaths and an equal number of serious heart damage. The nearly billion-dollar fine is in addition to hundreds of millions of dollars paid to injured patients and families.

The fact that any company could possibly be partially at fault for 50,000 dead people, and still be in business, makes us want to vomit.

Eli Lilly
Fine: $1,400,000,000
Year: 2009
Drug involved: *Zyprexa*, an antipsychotic
Criminal charges filed? Yes
Eli Lilly marketed this drug for conditions and patients — including the elderly and young children — for which it had not been determined safe. They also made dosage recommendations to doctors that were dangerous. Neither did Lilly appropriately reveal the side effects. Still in business.

Abbott
Fine: $1,500,000,000
Year: 2012
Drug involved: The mood stabilizer and antiepileptic *Depakote*
Criminal charges filed? Yes

Abbott illegally marketed Depakote as a treatment for combative dementia patients and schizophrenia, in spite of the fact that it wasn't approved for those conditions and resulted in severe side effects like anorexia. Still making pills.

Johnson & Johnson
Fine: $2,200,000,000
Year of settlement: 2012
Drugs involved: *Risperdal* and *Invega*, antipsychotics; *Natrecor*, a heart medication
Criminal charges filed? Yes

J&J's antipsychotic drugs were heavily marketed to child psychiatrists and physicians treating the elderly, in spite of the known side effects. The company hid data regarding the drugs' link to weight gain and diabetes. In the 1990s, J&J also funded the writing of a set of national treatment guidelines, the Texas Medical Algorithm Project, that were not based on valid information. Guidelines for the treatment of attention deficit hyperactivity disorder in children included Risperdal; however, the *FDA* never approved Risperdal for the treatment of ADHD, nor is there any evidence that it helps children with the condition. J & J had been investigated for nearly a decade for numerous violations, including secret payoffs to doctors on the take, and hiding what it knew were serious side effects to patients, They were sued by their own shareholders in 2010 for continued illegal business practices from the early 1990's.

In the normal world one might suspect their reputation to tarnish a bit. By now you know health care ain't a normal world. After a $2,200,000,000 fine, Johnson & Johnson was awarded "the world's most respected company" by *Barron's' Magazine* in 2008.

UN-believable.

GlaxoSmithKline
Fine: $3,000,000,000
Year: 2012
Drugs involved: *Paxil* and *Wellbutrin*, antidepressants; *Lamictal*, an antiepileptic
Criminal charges filed? Yes

GlaxoSmithKline's marketing crimes included promoting its drugs for unapproved uses; hiding data about medication risks; payoffs and lavish gifts, such as all-expenses-paid vacations to physicians. One of those involved was television's Doctor Drew, who apparently received $275,000 to promote Wellbutrin as a remedy for sexual dysfunction in depression, despite a lack of data on its use for that purpose. He did not disclose his payment from the company when he discussed the drug on his program.

❖

"The truth is that researchers have never discovered a single defective gene or accurately identified any chemical imbalance that

has caused an emotional disorder; nor have they ever proven that brain abnormalities are responsible for even one emotional disorder. In fact, the *National Institute of Mental Health* openly admits that the causes of schizophrenia, depression, mania, anxiety and hyperactivity are unknown."
Ty Colbert, MD
Author, Broken Brains or Wounded Hearts

❖

"I have become a very angry man. I've just realized that for 25 years I had been making my patients sick and big pharma rich. I've just realized that those chronic hepatitis patients that died waiting for a liver transplant could have been easily cured with vitamin C. I realize now that my toximolecular medical education only led me to do more harm than good."
Edward Cichowicz MD

❖

Interesting. There are no lab tests for psychiatry. No full-color printouts to verify who is sick and who is well. No EEG graph to prove who is sane and who is not. *The Diagnostic and Statistical Manual of Mental Disorders* – the *DSM* – is affectionately referred to as the Bible of psychiatric assessment. The *DSM* was originally printed in 1952 and has undergone a number of revisions over the last half-century. But Doctor Allen Frances, editor of the 4th edition of the psychiatric Bible, says it has also spawned some truly awful unintended consequences. Frances has been called "the most powerful psychiatrist in America" by *The New York Times*. But after decades of a career which placed him throat-deep in psychiatry, he has experienced an epiphany. He now believes the *DSM-IV* has contributed to over-treatment, over-medication, diagnostic exaggeration and psychiatric fashion. He is convinced the most recent edition threatens to turn everyday living into psychiatric disease. Frances' new book, *Saving Normal,* focuses on what's gone wrong, and how his profession might reel in psychiatry and the pharmaceutical assault.

His grim admission regarding the psychiatric Bible? *"We made mistakes that had terrible consequences."*

Here's a frightening example, he says, that connects the *American Psychiatric Association* with the epidemic of bipolar diagnoses in children over the past decade:

"Immediately after our book was published, doctors began to diagnose children as 'bipolar' even if they had never experienced a manic episode and were too young to have shown the necessary pattern of mood change. Within a decade, bipolar diagnoses among children had increased 4000%. Many of these kids were put on antipsychotic drugs, whose effects on the developing brain are poorly understood but which are known to cause obesity and diabetes."

In 2007 an investigation revealed that an influential advocate for diagnosing bipolar disorder in kids, *Harvard* psychiatrist Joseph Biederman, had neglected to tell anybody he had been paid $1,600,000 by Johnson & Johnson, makers of the bipolar drug Risperdal. Biederman had told the company his proposed trial of Risperdal in young children, "will support the safety and effectiveness of risperidone in this age group."

Biederman, considered by many to be the poster boy for marketing-based medicine, had been under investigation for two years. Doctor Frances now believes that America's 'bipolar fad' would not exist, had his *DSM-IV* committee agreed to limit the diagnosis to adults only, as was believed prudent at the time. He is certain the *DSM-IV* manual inadvertently caused faulty diagnoses of autism, attention-deficit hyperactivity disorder and bipolar disorder. He maintains the book encouraged the clinical tendency to chalk up life's difficulties to mental illness – and then treat them with drugs.

He observes that he had already regretted remaining silent when, in the 1980s, he watched the pharmaceutical industry insinuate itself into the *American Psychiatric Association's* training programs. Multi-million dollar drug company contributions to those programs continued annually until 2008, when the *APA* finally decided to phase out industry-supported education.

But the more that doctors reading the *DSM-IV* decided their patients were mentally ill and in need of drugs, the happier drug companies were.

A 2006 *University of Massachusetts* study found that over half of 170 psychiatric "experts" who helped work on the latest edition of the *DSM* had financial links to drug makers from 1989-1994, when the most recent edition was published. Those "financial links" included ownership of drug company stocks; travel expenses; research funding; consulting fees and cash payments.

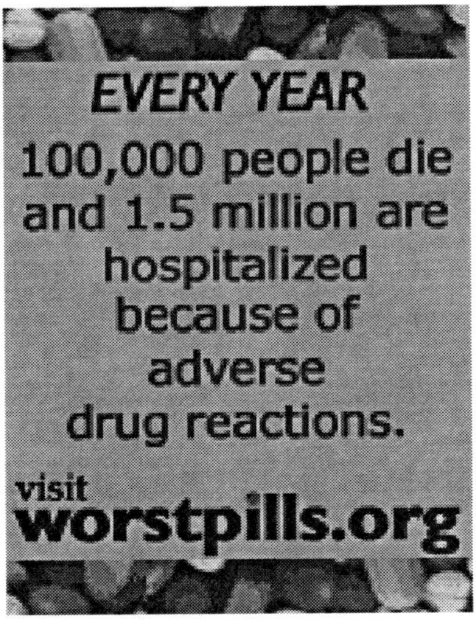
EVERY YEAR
100,000 people die
and 1.5 million are
hospitalized
because of
adverse
drug reactions.
visit
worstpills.org

Are your drugs in here? Don't you think you ought to check?

Want more nifty news? All of the experts involved in the *DSM* writings that define mood disorders, psychotic reactions and schizophrenia, were paid to say what they did. The fact that diseases can be invented – or as with homosexuality, *un*-invented – and their criteria altered in response to social whim, is exactly what worries Doctor Frances about some 'diagnoses,' such as Temper Dysregulation Disorder; Attenuated Psychotic Syndrome; Binge Eating Disorder, to name a few. He warns that the new *DSM-V*, with its emphasis on early intervention, will result in a "wholesale medicalization of normality" and "a bonanza for the pharmaceutical industry" for which patients would pay the "high price of adverse effects, dollars, and stigma."

He ends with this warning:

"This gives drug makers a new target for their hard sell and doctors, most of whom see it as part of their job to write prescriptions, even more reason to medicate."

❖

Here is what a basic drug study summary looks like:

Morbidity and mortality from medical errors: an increasingly serious public health problem

Phillips DP, Bredder CC.

Source
Department of Sociology, *University of California at San Diego, La Jolla*, California 92093, USA. dphillip@weber.ucsd.edu

Abstract
From 1983 to 1998, U.S. fatalities from acknowledged prescription errors increased by 243%, from 2,876 to 9,856 per year. This percentage increase is greater than for almost any other cause of death, and far outpaced the increase in the number of prescriptions. Many nonfatal prescription errors also occur, but estimates of the frequency of these errors vary widely, because various definitions, geographic settings, and institutions have been used. Efforts to reduce fatal and nonfatal prescription errors have encountered perceptual, legal, medical, and cultural barriers. It may be possible to reduce prescription errors by instituting a central agency responsible for collecting, analyzing, and reporting harmful or potentially harmful drug events, and for issuing recommendations and directives.

❖

Drug Recall due to safety issues 1980 – 2011

Here is a list of prescription drugs originally approved by the *Food & Drug Administration* as safe and effective. They were then pulled from the market when it turned out they were not safe after all. From 1973-1991, sixteen drugs were found to be too dangerous for use. Over the next 19 years, 28 more lethal drugs were withdrawn. Between the dates listed, hundreds of millions of doses were taken, just like doctors ordered. My partners and

I used to find some of these poor souls lying in the kitchen, as cold as the floor.

Drug	Approved/Disapproved
Methaqualone	1965/1982
Fenfluramine	1973/1997
Pemoline	1975/2005
Darvon/Darvocet	1976/2010
Ticrynafen	1979/1982
Zomax	1980/1983
Oraflex/Opren	1982/1982
Zimelidine	1982/1983
Halcyon	1982/1991
Nomifensine	1984/1986
Suprofen	1985/1987
Seldane	1985/1998
Etretinate	1986/1999
Encainide	1986/1991
Terodiline	1986/1991
Permax	1988/2007
Hismanal	1988/1999
Permax	1988/2007
Manoplax	1992/1993
Teflox	1992/1992
Propulsid	1993/2000
Orlaam	1993/2003
Aprotinin	1993/2007
Serelect	1995/1998
Redux	1996/1997
Duract	1997/1998
Raxar	1997/1999
Posicor	1997/1998
Baycol	1997/2001
Reductil/Meridia	1997/2010
Trovan	1997/2002
Avandia	1999/2010

Rezulin	1999/2000
Raplon	1999/2001
Vioxx	1999/2004
Tequin	1999/2006
Lotronex	2000/2000
Mylotarg	2000/2010
Xigris	2002/2011

❖

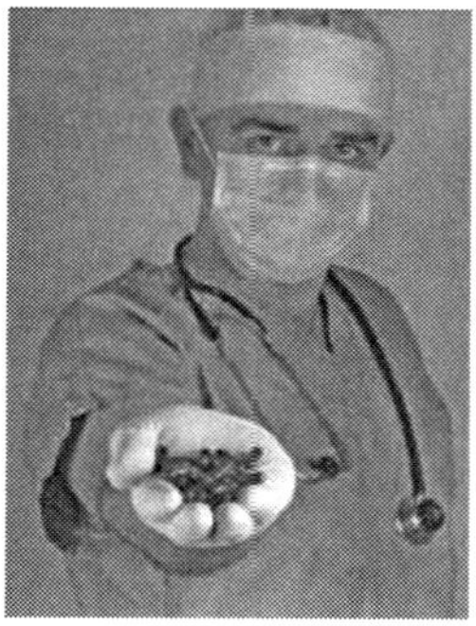

Trust me. I'm a doctor.

In ancient Athens the voting public would scratch the name of the desired outcast into a shard of stone and toss it into a circle in the soil. With enough votes counted, that person would then be banished from society. In a wiser future, we suspect the drug industry will face an equal banishment, its tally also etched into stone – the tombstones of the dead. We give it another hundred years.

❖

It is trendy to think of pill-popping as a form of optimism. Take these like M& Ms and good health will be yours. We slowly came to see non-emergent pharmaceuticals as the substrata for pessimism – because the drug-gobbling never stops. The cartels hold out 'good health' just beyond your reach – like the artificial rabbit at a dog race. The drug schemers hit their most profound home run in the 1970's, once they realized precisely how to defeat ethical resistance. They learned to simply maintain a callous disinterest in the millions they destroy, while yammering from the belfry about the thousands they help.

❖

"It is simply no longer possible to believe much of the clinical research that is published, or to rely on the judgment of trusted physicians or authoritative medical guidelines. I take no

pleasure in this conclusion, which I reached slowly and reluctantly over my two decades as an editor of *The New England Journal of Medicine*."
Doctor Marcia Angell
Harvard Medical School
Author, the Truth about Drug Companies: How They Deceive Us

We suggest you take a good, hard look at who is making this almost unbelievable statement. Marcia Angell is no kook on a street corner.

❖

And so it came to pass that Henry W. Gadsden, Chief Executive Officer of Merck from 1965 to 1975, was the madman at the helm during that drug giant's massive rise to power. Here was a freak who ought to have left his brain to science fiction. He saw to it that their expenditures for research and development jumped 400% - from $32,000,000 a year to $125,000,000. Merck's revenues exceeded $1,000,000,000 for the first time that decade.

Under his direction, Merck defined the target of the entire pharmaceutical tsunami by the mid-1970s: **Everybody**. From that point forward, they would adopt the marketing tactics that cosmetics were already using so successfully. They would employ psychological weapons to exploit citizen fears of illness; fretting over physical appearance flaws; doubting their sexual performance; appalled at the thought of aging. Have an excitable kid? Not a problem. We've got pills for that. With his stated plan to sell drugs like "chewing gum" a leviathan was spawned, and with it a colossal energy that injures and kills and bankrupts its way through a largely ignorant, extremely gullible society. It convinces people of good health that they are unwell, by counting on our intellectual sluggishness.

Merck saw even more wealth on the horizon by taking physicians out of the marketing equation, at least in part. They started the first-ever 'direct-to-consumer' ads in the *Reader's Digest* in 1981. Television propaganda rapidly followed. There

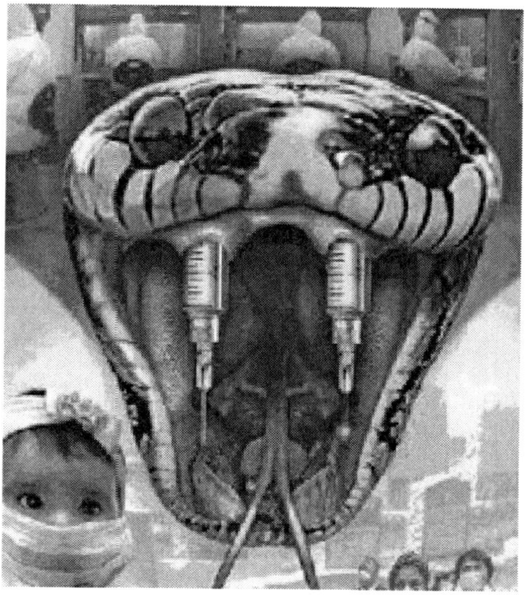

Go ahead. Make my day.

was gold to be mined from societal paranoia, as long as they kept stirring the pot. These unconscionable ploys methodically perfected the formula to seduce practically every man and woman, and children at the earliest possible ages. What a glorious achievement of modern America. A rapt clientele of millions hooked on drugs – paying customers for life.

And to think our citizenry actually believes these poisons are a whole sight better than Wrigley's chewing gum, is rather ironic. Gum tastes great, calms the nerves, staves overeating and kills practically nobody.

Immutable Law #8

Health care is joined at the spleen to the most rabid drug cartels on the planet. This betrothal destroys as many lives as it saves. And we in EMS are your fast-track through the front door.

Modern version of the Hippocratic Oath

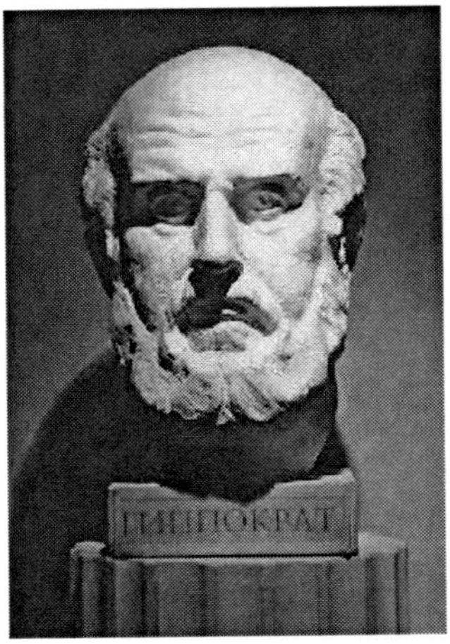

"I swear to fulfill, to the best of my ability and judgment, this covenant:

I will respect the hard-won scientific gains of those physicians in whose steps I walk and gladly share such knowledge as is mine with those who follow.

I will apply, for the benefit of the sick, all measures required, avoiding those twin traps of overtreatment and therapeutic nihilism.

"Whenever a doctor cannot do good, he must be kept from doing harm."

—Hippocrates of Cos

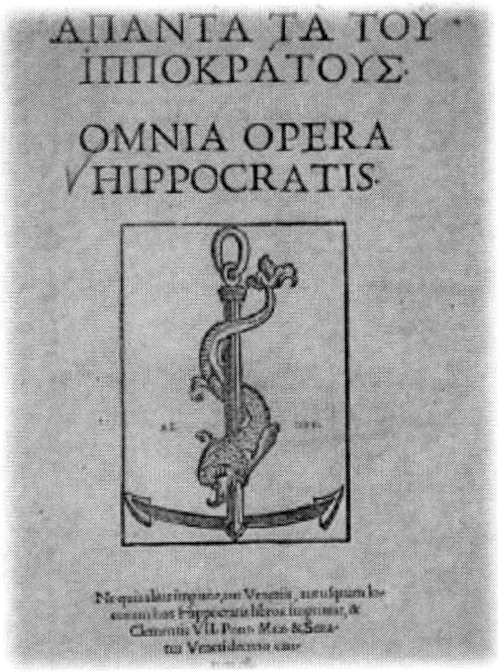

ΑΠΑΝΤΑ ΤΑ ΤΟΥ ΙΠΠΟΚΡΑΤΟΥΣ·

OMNIA OPERA HIPPOCRATIS·

I will remember there is art to medicine as well as science, and that warmth, sympathy, and understanding may outweigh the surgeon's knife or the chemist's drug.

I will not be ashamed to say 'I know not,' nor will I fail to call in my colleagues when the skills of another are needed for a patient's recovery.

I will respect the privacy of my patients, for their problems are not disclosed to me that the world may know.

Most especially must I tread with care in matters of life and death. If it is given me to save a life, all thanks. But it may also be within my power to take a life; this awesome responsibility must be faced with great humbleness and awareness of my own frailty. Above all, I must not play at God.

I will remember that I do not treat a fever chart, a cancerous growth, but a sick human being, whose illness may affect the person's family and economic stability. My responsibility includes these related problems, if I am to care adequately for the sick.

I will prevent disease whenever I can, for prevention is preferable to cure.

I will remember that I remain a member of society, with special obligations to all my fellow human beings, those sound of mind and body as well as the infirm.

If I do not violate this oath, may I enjoy life and art, respected while I live and remembered with affection thereafter. May I always act so as to preserve the finest traditions of my calling and may I long experience the joy of healing those who seek my help."

Hippocrates, generally referred to as the Father of Modern Medicine, is believed to have been born 450 years before the Nazarene, on the Greek island of Cos. He was a physician who lived during the Classical era of Greece and founded a medical school based upon what were at the time rather unique ideas on biomedical observations and causes and treatments of disease. He was one of the first physicians known to have strongly proposed a highly ethical approach to the profession.

Unfortunately it is almost impossible to separate the reality of Hippocrates' life from the parables surrounding him over centuries gone by. About fifty original documents exist today with his name on them, but almost none could have been written by him. The most famous, of course, is the Hippocratic Oath which – most historians concur – he certainly did not write. The Oath does – it is believed – accurately sum up the philosophy by which he lived.

"Doctors kill 680 people ever day of the year in this country. Imagine if two jumbo jets started crashing every day, killing 4,760 passengers a week. How many weeks do you think would go by before we started grounding airliners? One? Not even."

—Barbara Starfield, MD
Researcher, Author
Distinguished Professor
Johns Hopkins University

What do you suppose Hippocrates would say to this?

Chapter Nine

There are variables, like where you live and how you live. But the typical citizen walking in the mall is far more likely to be killed by a physician than by a homicidal maniac with a gun.

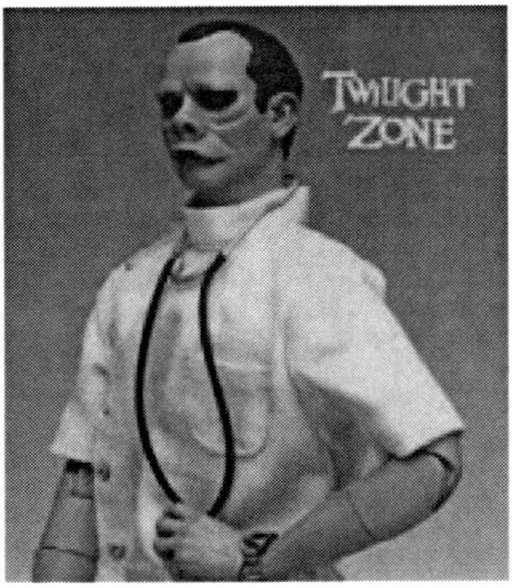

Oh, they can fool anybody from a distance

I was not even out of school before I witnessed my first doctor commit murder. It would not be my last – Lord, no – but I can recall that night as vividly as though it happened last week. Few medics forget their first physician homicide.

It happened in what we called "phase-three," the final aspect of the program triad that follows classroom and then clinical rotations. Phase-three is field internship, where the student-medic eats, sleeps, works and breathes with two veteran medic trainers, 24-hours at a time. My particular field training was an assignment at *Solana Beach Fire*, on the North Coast of San Diego County. Solana Beach was one of the first medic teams in California, and its group of six were 30-40 year-old medics who knew what they were doing. From shoreline and freeways to lagoons and cliff-tops, they pretty much experienced everything the world of rescue had to offer, and they saw it six times a day. But until this night, they had never seen one like this.

Within our response area lay a breathtakingly wealthy community known as Rancho Santa Fe, a few miles inland, and the 911 call came in as an "unconscious female." We piled into the ambulance late one cold February evening and within 10 minutes located the correct address. It was a tiled-roof, Mediterranean-style masterpiece surrounded by a garden of marvelous landscape. We entered the home through the foyer, found ourselves in the well-lit dining room, and that was where the curiosities started piling up. The dinner table was the strangest we'd ever seen: maybe three feet wide; nearly a foot thick; probably twenty feet long – a massive chunk of polished lumber. A gold plaque on its base proclaimed that it was made of something called African Mahogany-Carpathian Elm meld; that it was once the keel of a 500 year-old British warship, the *Little Barbara of Greenwich*. Wow. At the far end of the table sat a trim, dark-haired fellow who managed formality even in his casual wear. He looked to be in his mid-fifties. Standing at attention to his right was a manservant with a white cloth draped over his forearm. At the empty end of the table we could see a plate of half-eaten food, supervised by a woman servant with her own cloth.

The gentleman of the house spoke calmly as he chewed his steak. "My wife's gone off down the hall to her room. She's thrown another tiresome snit."

We located the woman sprawled diagonally across a large bed, head facing away from us. Her face was well into the pillow. I made eye contact with my primary trainer, Jeff, whose nod meant they wanted me to direct the rescue procedures. In field training it does not matter that the veteran medics can care for a dying woman quicker than an intern. Rescue is on-the-job-training. I checked quickly for any sign of trauma and then had somebody help me roll her over. Lying on her back, it was easy to see the foam oozing from her mouth, so we got her onto her side and started clearing her airway. Surrounding her on the bed were empty pill bottles, and I had a partner read them off to me as I applied oxygen to the woman and prepped her arm for an IV.

"Looks like she's loaded up with benzodiazepines, antihistamines and melatonin," a voice behind me said. "Looks like half a bottle of Vodka is gone, too."

At some point I became aware of a fire crew gathering in the hallway behind us. I opened her blouse and applied three EKG electrodes to triangulate the heart. I'd already injected two doses of naloxone into her veins, but did not expect it to help on non-narcotic depressants. Her pupils were large and relaxed – not pinpoint as in narcotic ODs. My patient was 54, with a tussle of short brown hair and slack expression. And within two minutes we all knew that even though she had a normal heart rhythm, a decent pulse and blood pressure, she was not going to breathe on her own.

"Bag her and go?" a firefighter asked, to which I answered, "Absolutely."

Although scenes such as this appear stressful to the onlooker, our patient presented no challenge at all. An unconscious adult puts up no fight whatsoever, and with a bag/mask and oxygen, we could breathe better for her than she could for herself. With the IV in place we could now administer any emergency drug she might need, should her heart begin to sputter. At the hospital they would switch our IV to a saline drip and hook her up to an automatic breathing machine. Most likely she'd wake up tomorrow healthy enough to have lunch in bed. And *Scripps Memorial* had darned good food.

As we rolled the gurney slowly through the dining room I have such a clear memory of the stunned look on the husband's face. I know I will never forget what he said into the phone. "My God, she's alive. They're taking her. You'd better get over here."

None of us knew what that meant, so we worked our way out the door, across cobblestone and were just prepping to put her into the ambulance when a glossy black Jaguar came sliding into the gravel drive and skidded to a stop. The ambulance lights lit up a scene that must have looked like a movie.

The driver of the Jaguar exited quickly and spoke out to us. "I'm Doctor Gary Ernstein and this woman is my patient. I appreciate your care but I need you to return her to her bedroom and I'll take over from there."

Well, you could have heard a catheter drop because this just did not happen. On those rare cases where MDs happen upon emergency scenes, they generally stay completely out of the Paramedics' way. This may seem odd to you of normal mind but the reality is, few doctors have better than a vague idea how to manage an emergency. If the patient happens to be theirs, following along behind us is by far the wiser choice, so that's what many of them do.

But not Jaguar-man.

My preceptor Jeff stepped forward. "Doctor Ernstein, this woman is not breathing. The rest of her vital signs are within normal limits, but whatever she took has knocked out her respiratory drive."

"I understand," Ernstein said. "But I'll take it from here. Please put her back in the house."

"Do you have any respiratory equipment with you, Sir?"

We all knew that he didn't and even if he did, was his plan to sit on the edge of her bed and breathe for her all night?

"I have what I need. Put her back in her room."

As the incident played out I glanced back at the house, to see the husband standing at the window watching the drama in the driveway. By all indications the honeymoon was over.

Veteran medic Jeff was gritting his teeth tight enough to bunch up his jaw muscles. He flipped on the field radio and reached the base hospital ER. He put the radio on speaker-phone so that we all could hear. The night crackled with the sudden voice of the physician on duty. Jeff gave him a quick rundown of the situation. Confident that no base hospital on the planet would allow an unconscious patient to be returned to a bedroom, we all waited for the ER doctor to advise Jaguar-man that what he wanted to do was not in the patient's best interest.

Incredibly, the base physician came back with this: "I know it's a tough spot, Jeff. But we've checked and Doctor Ernstein is the MD of record for the patient. So we need to acquiesce to his best judgment."

Firefighters looked around at each other incredulously. Jeff flashed an expression of anger, but he was the consummate pro and answered the ER physician without yelling. "She's . . . not . . . breathing. She needs intubation and a respirator. She's going to die in the bed."

The brief silence at the end of the line was almost palpable. "I understand your concern. We need to let Doctor Ernstein take over her care."

So we wheeled the comatose woman back to her bedroom, disconnected her lifelines, left the house and drove away.

Four days later we were starting a new shift at *Solana Beach Fire*. We sat around the big kitchen table, sipping coffee from cups that sported comments like, 'I'm not deaf . . . I'm ignoring you.' We cracked the first goofy jokes of the day. That was when the fire captain slid a folded newspaper over to us, and we all gaped at the small headline on page five:

Barbara Lucille Martin-Greenwald Passes Away
Auto Heiress Found Dead of Natural Causes

(*San Diego Union* obituary)

So the husband wanted her dead. He knew he could provoke her into an overdose because he had probably done it before. The doctor-buddy went along with the program for reasons we can only surmise. That's all it takes really, for a razor-sharp conspiracy in the health care biz. There would be no autopsy to reveal something sinister, say, in the liquor; no questioning of the husband on the little matter of her face being so deeply into the pillow

– not with a pecksniffian MD willing to falsify a death certificate. That's a 60-second chat on the phone with the coroner. Some like to say there is no such thing as a perfect murder. You will never hear an experienced Paramedic say that. This was the *perfect* murder. Guess who got that fine house and that cool dining room table carved right out of a boat's butt – out in Rancho Santa Fe? Life at its finest, bankrolled by the dead auto heiress, now out of the way. End of story.

Any questions?

❖

Those of feeble capacities often parrot that outrageous physician misbehavior – as the case noted above – is a rare event. Au contraire. By the time you finish this chapter you, at least, will be properly informed:

Martin MacNeill MD, Utah – Prison, Murder of wife by drugging, drowning

Conrad Murray MD, L.A. – Guilty, Manslaughter, Michael Jackson

Clara Harris DDS, Houston – Prison, "Murder by Mercedes" death of her philandering husband, also a physician

Ronald Mikos MD, Illinois – Life-term, Murder of patient who was about to testify against him

Harry Sugar MD, New York – Life-term, Murder of wife Joan

George Kubski MD, Florida – 20-year term, prescribing 20,000 narcotic doses in 90 days; O.D. death of a patient

Michael Posey DDS, Napa CA – Prison, Murder of wife Elizabeth

Robert Weitzel MD, Utah – 15-year sentence, narcotic deaths of five elderly patients

Barton Corbin DDS, Atlanta – Life-term, Murder, wife (recently) Murder, girlfriend (many years ago)

Charles E. Friedgood MD, NY – Life-term, Murder of his wife Sophie, injection overdose

❖

Physician arrogance is birthed when a narcissistic mind slips on a lab coat. And heaping praise and money upon these people is just about as bright as tossing the car keys and a beer to a teenager.

❖

Dirk Greineder MD, New England – Life-term, Murder of wife with a hammer

Robert Bierenbaum MD, NY – Life-term, Murder, Dismemberment, wife Gail; body tossed from airplane

Harriston Bass MD, Las Vegas – 25-year term, Murder by overdose

Richard Sharp MD, Boston – Found hanged in prison cell, serving time For Murder, his wife

Bradley Schwartz MD, Tucson – Prison for Murder

John B Hamilton MD, OK City – Life-term, Murder of his wife

Carl Drury MD, Georgia – 15-year term, plot to Murder his wife

John D Cavaness MD, Illinois – Death Row, Murder of his son

Thomas G Merrill MD, Florida – Life-term, overdosing patients, 5 deaths

❖

It was three years later and we were assigned to Fire Station #17 in East San Diego. My partner and I were operating in one of the busiest EMS service zones in California, averaging 128 responses each month. And that was just our tally on "C" shift. "A" and "B" shifts were doing the same crazy thing.

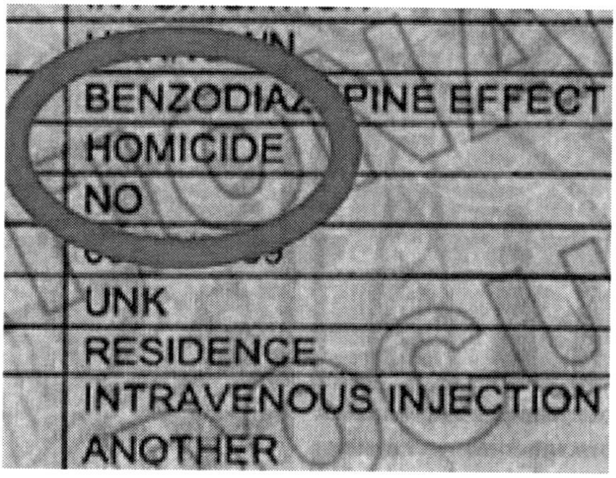

Now, one of the true perks of EMS is that we rarely see the same patients twice, so even if they get on your nerves – and plenty of them do – we take comfort in knowing they will be out of our lives in less than an hour. Pity, but the same cannot be said for physicians who kill patients, because if you happen to have a "Double-Oh-Doc" in your service area (Like James Bond, they get paychecks after killing people) you are going to deal with him over and over.

We say "him" because none of us have ever known a lady Double-Oh. Fascinating, that. The 2% lunatic fringe keeps right on rolling along, day after day, year after year. One of the little known facts of medicine is that when the excrement hits the fan at a doctor's office, they call Paramedics to solve the problem. They say it happens just over 40 times an hour in this country.

In East San Diego we had three Double-Oh's that we knew about, churning out garbage-level patient care, one case at a time. But the most prolific was a dentist named Raf Coronado. Time after time Coronado, age 51, would ignore his nurses' warnings pointing out patient allergies. And these warnings were not exactly hidden. They were written in large print on the medical files and highlighted in yellow. Allergic to Lidocaine. We guessed any citizen smarter than a 5th grader could probably figure it out. Not this draftsack. He gave Lidocaine to everybody. Why? "It's a wonderful drug. My favorite drug," he'd say, even as we worked to retrieve another patient on the floor of his office. "I know what I'm doing."

Really.

We knew what he was doing, too. And we knew what we were doing. We were repeatedly wrenching some poor soul from the jaws of a Third World Assassin. Sometimes it worked. Sometimes it didn't. By our count, clinical cretin Coronado killed at least three patients in the early 1980s alone, and did his best to kill seven others.

Did we write reports to the *California State Medical Board* begging for an investigation of this medical muttonhead? Numerous times. Were we interviewed by San Diego homicide detectives? More than once.

Was he ever punished?

Not even close. Coronado retired a gleeful, wealthy man; moved to Mazatlan and died on a yacht while eating a shrimp salad with a prostitute 27 years ago.

America. What a country. Ole!

❖

There was a time when communities could shame their doctors into better behavior. Those days are over.

❖

Mark Benson MD, Michigan – 30-year term, DUI crash kills family of 3

David W Webb MD, Florida – Life sentence, 130 counts, illegal drug dealing, four patient deaths

Ehigiator Akhigbe MD, Wash DC – Health Care Fraud, 'Ghost Visits'

Sumit Sinha MD, Wisconsin – Fired, taking wife & child on Christmas shoplifting spree at Macy's

Kevin Lickfield MD, Penn – Guilty, treating patients after license revocation. Third conviction in 10 years

Lewis Jackson MD, Georgia – Guilty, Patient Sexual Assault in prison

Craig Bittner MD, L.A. – Fled the country, using human body fat for SUV fuel

Lesley M. Scholl MD, Indiana – Guilty, Murder plot, his wife & 2 others

Adam Lokeh MD, MN – Medical Board sanctions, falsifying prescriptions

David C. Winkler MD, Texas – Prison, Child Pornography

Brian J. McDevitt MD, WV – Convicted, Illegal Distribution of Drugs

Bruce S. Smith MD, Chicago – 18-years, Rape, his pregnant patient

John D. Kristofic MD, PA – Guilty, $1,000,000 Medical Fraud

Stephen Grandstaff MD, AL – Prison, 73 counts, Drugs-for-Sex case

Ahmed Rashed MD, NJ – Guilty, Theft of a Human Body Part, stole a hand to impress a topless dancer

❖

Private school medical director admits guilt in child porn case

A physician employed by the elite *Phillips Academy* in Andover Massachusetts has been convicted on child pornography charges.

Doctor Richard Keller, age 57, the former medical director at the prestigious school for nearly 20 years, admitted to purchasing between 50-100 DVDs from a Canadian video source. Nearly all of the images, according to prosecutors, were of young boys engaging in sexual activity.

Investigators learned that Keller had been reprimanded as far back as 1999 for using the academy's health center computer to access pornography. He was also warned to stop showing sexually explicit cartoons to students 10 years ago. As is typical with physicians, he was never seriously sanctioned.

Keller, who worked with juvenile patients as a pediatric endocrinologist at *Children's Hospital* in Boston and taught at *Harvard Medical School*, will reside in a Massachusetts state prison for the next six years.

❖

David L. Hoban MD, CA – Chief Psychiatrist, Salinas Valley Prison, Guilty, $40,000 Time Card Embezzlement

Carl Bergstrom MD, Carmel CA – Guilty, Sexual Assault

Kentrell Liddell MD, MS – Chief Medical Officer of the State Prison, Guilty, $94,000 Embezzlement

❖

The physician population in this country does not need better oversight. It needs an exorcism.

❖

George S. Kooshian MD, L.A. – Guilty, diluting AIDS patients' medications

Michael Kim MD, Houston – Guilty, "pill mill" operation, 2,000,000 doses of hydrocodone; defrauded Medicare of $1.7 million

David W. Webb MD, PA – Guilty, 36 counts of Fraud; Illegal Drug Distribution; ID Theft

Rees G. Freeman MD, OR – License Revoked, Incompetency

Mark J. Baskerville MD, OR – License Suspended, Repeated Drug Use

John P. Guereiro MD, OR – State Corrective Action, inappropriate behavior during female patient exams

Fred A. Hogan MD, Michigan – Guilty, Illegal Drug Prescription, Medical Records Falsification

Jeffrey A. Luty MD, Portland – Oregon State Medical License Revoked

Russell Reitz MD, Topeka, KS – Guilty, Aggravated Assault & Battery

Kevin M. Denney MD, Tampa – Guilty, Illegal Drug Prescriptions

Ana A. Jacinto MD, Florida – Guilty, HIV Infusion Fraud, $11 million scam. Sentenced to 30 years

David D. Campbell MD, Oregon – Per State Order - may no longer examine female patients

Phillip Astin MD, Georgia – Physician of pro wrestler Chris Benoit, Guilty, 175 counts illegal drug prescriptions to known drug abusers

Steven B. Schwartz MD, SD – License Revoked; 30 malpractice lawsuits

❖

We had not even started using our new stethoscopes in school yet when we came face to face with the homicidal doctor reality. Had we considered the subject at all prior to school, we would have surmised what many folks do – that sure sometimes, in the high-wire act of lifesaving, mistakes happen. Trust us. We would not waste the energy writing a book focused merely on medical errors. Of course they happen and they happen every day. And many times when people die it simply has nothing to do with ill will at all.

On the other hand, here in the *Twilight Zone*, it often does:

One morning in our first month we showed up for class to find this note on the door, written by our primary instructor:

"You can take a break until 9:00. Our neurotrauma lecturer has a pressing legal matter and won't be joining us today."

Well, our neurotrauma lecturer turned out to be Doctor Jeffrey MacDonald, ER director at *St. Mary's Medical Center* in Long Beach. And the pressing legal matter? He was about to be convicted of chopping up his wife and two baby girls. And a baby boy, if you count the one in Collette's womb.

Background on the infamous Jeffrey Robert MacDonald murder case can easily be found elsewhere, and we see no reason to go into detail here. Suffice it to say that one of the most popular medical instructors in Southern California is still in prison for butchering his pregnant wife and two little blond daughters. We were a chatty bunch left speechless. Novitiates all, we were just opening our naïve little minds. And what were we seeing? Well, damn it, physicians around us were killing people – both in and out of their lab coats. And when you're young and wide-eyed and guileless, that's a little unsettling.

❖

Joel Bernstein MD, San Diego – Probation, Unapproved Cancer Drugs

Nimesh Patel MD, WA – Guilty, Fine, kickback scheme

Shashi Agarwal MD, NJ – Prison, MRI kickback scheme

Stephen Bossenberry MD, MI – License Suspended, Domestic Violence

Frank Lobacz MD, Chicago – Sentenced, 5 years, Health Care Fraud

Timothy J. Palmer D.O. GA – Medical License Revoked

Roger Hershline MD, SC – Prison, Dealing Narcotics

Carlos Bray, MD, Indiana – License Surrender, Incompetence

Jon S. Opsahl MD, CA – Guilty, Drug misbranding

Ramon E. Ravelo MD, NY – Settled, $2M Sexual Harassment suit

Kenneth Mudd MD, Kentucky – Prison, selling blank prescription pads

Mukundha Mukerjee MD, Mich – Sentenced, 328 years, Drug Trafficking

Elizabeth Reimers MD, Tenn – Convicted, Illegal Narcotic Dispensing

❖

Bad physicians get little attention until it is far too late

The story of the modern-day medical monster Kermit Gosnell is just about as nauseating as anything to be found in medicine. It is a case about yet another MD with the 'God Complex' – one who took particular delight in butchering babies and injuring their mothers. As is typical in healthcare, many of this man's unspeakable antics were reported, but ignored by those in position to stop him, for years. Gosnell would on a nightly basis deliver live babies in the back rooms of his "clinic" and then sever their necks with scissors. The manner in which his clinic operated included appalling fraud; overdosing pregnant women with dangerous drugs; spreading venereal disease among them with infected instruments; perforating internal organs and killing people. This went on for decades.

Former employee Stephen Massof described during the trial how they would "snip the spinal chords" of babies, separating the brain from the body. He testified that at times, when women were given medicine to speed up their deliveries, "it would rain fetuses. Fetuses and blood all over the place.".

One former employee described hearing a baby screaming after it was delivered during an abortion procedure. "It sounded like a little alien," she said.

This former Philadelphia doctor was finally convicted of murder in 2013, and has been sentenced to two life terms. Gosnell, age 72, was facing the death penalty at the time of his plea agreement. He was convicted of numerous other felonies as well, including manslaughter, conspiracy and the operation of a corrupt business. Former clinic employees testified that Gosnell routinely delivered babies who were still breathing, moaning and moving. They reported that over the years, he and his assistants would kill the newborns by "snipping" their spines at the back of the neck. Then, just for fun, he would cut off their tiny feet and store them in refrigerated jars.

❖

Paul J. O'Brian D.O., Indiana – Guilty, Narcotic Possession by Fraud

Sanford K. Myers MD, Tenn. – Prison 13 years, Narcotic Distribution

Kenneth D. Richards D.O., MO – Guilty, possession drug paraphernalia

Louis Ortenzio MD, WV – Convicted, Health Care Fraud

Barry N. Odegaard MD, Hawaii – Prison, Narcotic Distribution

Nathan P. Stine MD, Spokane – Probation, 5 years, Illegal Prescriptions

Earl Sunderhaus MD, NC – License Suspension, shoving strangers in a store; poking female patients; cursing at members of the state medical board

Manuel B. Nigalan MD, NJ – Prison, Narcotic Distribution

Michael F Myers MD, SC – Prison, 30 counts, Narcotic Distribution

Cmdr Kevin Ronan MD, U.S. Navy – Federal Prison, filming sailor sex acts

Eric L. Ressner MD, Palm Beach – Guilty, Conspiracy to Commit Fraud

Scott McClelland MD, U.S. Navy – Guilty, Sex Solicitation, female patients

Breton L. Morgan MD, WV – Pled Guilty, Narcotics by Fraud

Yash Khanna MD, New Jersey – Convicted, medical lab kickback scheme

Christopher Card MD, Idaho – Convicted, Medicare Theft

Spurgeon Green Jr. MD, Georgia – 30-year term, Narcotic dealing

Bruce Jacobson MD, Wash. – Guilty, Child Pornography

Felix Rodriguez MD, Yonkers NY – Convicted, Narcotic Drug Ring

Samuel Bracken Jr, MD, Ohio – Guilty, oral sex with a child

Bradford Roberg MD, Illinois – Guilty, Forgery, faked a prescription of a dead patient for his personal use

Segun Rasaki MD, Indiana – Convicted, Patient Sexual Assault

Jayaram, MD, Trenton NJ – Guilty, Attempted Murder, a mistress he owed $250,000

❖

Sometimes the doctor homicides are downright vaudevillian. Grab a bag of pretzels, sit back and watch this one:

It was a typical weekend in Palm Springs. The hotels were full; the palm trees were blowing and the spirits were flowing. At the Riviera Resort – yes, the one where Elvis once seduced Mamie van Doren in a car on her honeymoon to somebody else – they had pulled out all the stops for an annual medical convention. According to the symposium banner, they were entertaining a distinguished crowd of 385. Our 911 call came in just after 7:30pm with the dispatcher telling us, "Adult male with chest pain."

We were half-way there already, at *Desert Hospital*, because that's where the peach pie was. So our response time to the Riviera was less than three minutes. En route we were updated that, "The patient is critical, now unconscious." We soon realized that getting across town in weekend traffic was not going to be the obstacle of the night. But navigating that last 100 feet into the ballroom was a task of Olympian proportions. Ask any medic and you'll get told that a doctor on-scene is not our favorite nightmare. There must exist a Euclidean formula in the universe. It dictates that a patient's proximity to survival, is inversely proportionate to the number of MDs in the room. Multiply that by 385 and you can appreciate the ugly math in this case.

We could see they had the patient on the carpeted floor, which was good, but they also had 10 dozen inebriated doctors around him, and that wasn't good at all. Well, to be fair, they weren't all doctors. About half in the crowd were pickled spouses in tight skirts, with a couple dozen call girls in the mix, just to spice things up. Tax write-offs for medical education are gleeful matters to behold. My partner recognized a few of the women, he said, and shouted out over the din that they flew in on contract from Las Vegas, complements of the medical conference organizers. I kept wondering how he knew all this. In the midst of the uproar we nodded and smiled at the professional ladies. Not only did they smell great but they were, after all, the most polite, least swacked people in the room.

We tried multiple times to run the gauntlet to the patient but there were just too many besozzled MDs to let that happen. We heard a dozen versions of, "Heyyy! Waht de hell! Ahm a ducktor, damn it!" Palm Springs police are an outstanding group, and upon arrival they immediately reacted to our predicament. They called for backup and started tossing drunks in fine clothing left and right. Six or eight of the degreed nutcases took indignant swings at the cops. That didn't go well. They ended up handcuffed and slammed to the carpet.

We edged closer to the man on his back, now in full-body seizure. Still too far away to do him any good at all, I glanced down at the defibrillator in my hand and wondered about the downside of shocking a few of these imbeciles between the ears. I honestly came close. It seemed appropriate to me. After a time we did get to the patient. By now he was in serious heart failure. All the while we were being poked and prodded, slapped and grabbed by the physicians around us. We did not dare open the drug box – these chimpanzees would have started grabbing at the needles. We eventually got him out of there, into the ambulance where we could think.

By our estimation he'd been 'down' at least 12 minutes and had no chance at all. Our EKG showed a rapidly dying heart. My partner breathed oxygen into the poor man while I infused our cocktail of atropine and epinephrine, sodium bicarbonate and calcium chloride. As we pulled slowly out of the parking lot I took a final peek at the Riviera medical convention, which inanely billed itself, "The Pinnacle of U.S. Health Care." Yes, it really did say that. It was a gathering to remember and I planned on savoring every detail. Through the rear window the last thing I spied was a highly-charged blond in tight black jumping onto the back of a Palm Springs cop, screaming that her, "Goddamned husband was a Goddamned cardiologist, Goddamn it!"

Her ballroom cardiologist had done this fellow no favors. What he and his colleagues did accomplish was something we had never quite witnessed: a collectively simian, 100% legal, group homicide. The man's name turned out to be Anthony Ward, a pharmaceutical sales rep. And Mr. Ward's death warrant was as good as signed the moment he sat down for prime rib surrounded by a hotel full of snockered doctors.

In the *Desert Hospital* chapel later that night we met briefly with Mr. Ward's grieving wife. She said through grateful tears that he was probably lucky that he had all those doctors in there helping him. I gritted my teeth hard enough to pulverize a molar. Her husband would have had better odds at a Cub Scout Jamboree. Those little guys are better organized; the worst they drink is Kool Aid, and they almost always know their merit badge limitations.

❖

A note worth mentioning: three months later a handful of cardiologists from the convention hired a law firm to sue my partner and me, as well as *Springs Ambulance Company*, for "interference of physician procedures during emergent patient care." They also filed a lawsuit against *Palm Springs Police Department*, citing "excessive force." Neither suit went anywhere. After a pair of depositions they simply disappeared. To this day I have no idea whether our sworn statements helped persuade those polished Chicago attorneys to drop the case or not. Because I was under oath, I observed that a doctor's wife leaping upon the back of an officer of the law seemed a little over the top. And I felt legally compelled to mention the exemplary behavior of the call girls. It was clear they had a calming effect on their highly intoxicated physician companions. Being sober, they would make excellent witnesses for the doctors. It's kind of fun to consider my sworn testimony may have dampened their enthusiasm for moving the case into a courtroom, so whether it did or not, I'll relish the thought a little while longer. You have got to admit it's a terrific mental image.

❖

Keith D. Goldblum MD, Ohio – 21-year term, Multiple Child Rape

Michael J. Milette MD, Illinois – Guilty, sold 62,000,000 doses of narcotics over the internet

Sarfraz A. Mirza MD, Florida – Convicted, Narcotic Trafficking

Tandy McElwee MD, LA – Prison, Narcotics Conspiracy

Carolyn McGrail MD, Florida – Pled Guilty, Health Care Fraud

Luis Molmenti MD, Mass – Convicted, Health Care Fraud

Michael Kamrava MD, Bev Hills – Guilty, Fertility Ethics, "Octo-mom" case

David Nash MD, Alabama – Convicted of Murder

Ronald A. McIver D.O., SC – 30-year term, Narcotics Distribution

John Rew MD, Tampa – Pleaded Guilty, Narcotic Distribution

Thomas Merrill D.O., Florida – Life term, Death of 5 patients due to illegal narcotic prescriptions

Richard Schlesinger MD, MD – Convicted, Health Care Fraud

Jack Voight MD, New Orleans – Guilty, Health Care Fraud, Conspiracy

Evelyn F. Sabugo MD, PA – Guilty, Conspiracy, Health Care Fraud

Kenneth J. Tolman MD – Convicted, Internet Solicitation of Sex with a 13-year old

Bernard Rottschaefer MD, PA – Prison, Narcotic Distribution

Thomas Bray MD, Bend OR – 25-years, Rape, Sodomy, Strangulation

❖

California MD gets 11 years for coffee shop drug-dealing

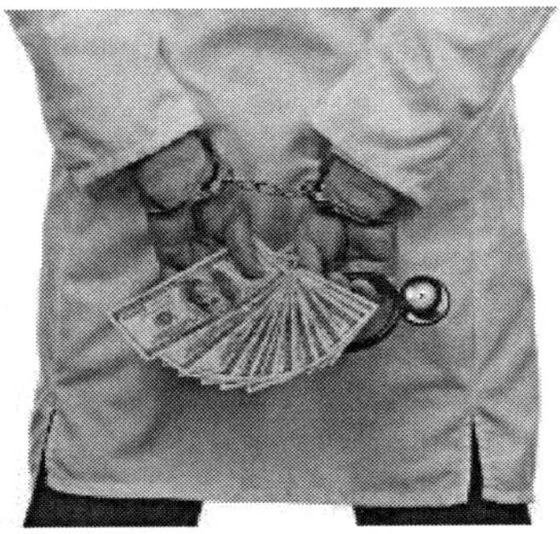

In our world we call it a "wallet biopsy"

A physician in Orange County has been sentenced to more than a decade in state prison for meeting "patients" at Starbucks coffee shops and prescribing narcotics after his 60-second chats.

Doctor Alvin Ming-Czech-Yee, age 44 of Mission Viejo, was told this at his sentencing: "You abused your position," U.S. District Judge Andrew Guilford said. "People came to you for healing and are worse for the experience."

Prosecutors revealed that Yee would meet people at various Starbucks throughout Orange County and that he charged as much as $600 in exchange for prescriptions for Xanex, Oxycontin and Vicoden. His 'examinations' lasted about a minute and consisted of checking pulses and blood pressures, and having people bend over to touch their toes.

According to detectives, at least two of Yee's so-called patients died of overdoses. As is typical, the drug-pusher was not charged in those deaths.

❖

Richard A. Mazur MD, MS – Prison, Narcotic Distribution

Can D. Phung MD, Okla. City – Serving 10-year term, narcotics charges

Lynn B. Pirie D.O., Phoenix – Guilty, Illegally Dispensing Human Growth Hormone

Jeffrey Pont MD, Scottsdale – Convicted, narcotics charge

Andrew Poulshock D.O., PA – Guilty, Drug Misbranding

John A. Petrovich MD, Illinois – Convicted, Health Care Fraud

Carlin G. Bartschi MD, AZ – Prison, multiple fraud felonies

Lawrence L. Parris MD, Wash. – Guilty, Unlawful Possession, Narcotics

David R. Bolick MD, Utah – Revocation of License; Bank Fraud

Paul Maynard MD, Virgin Is. – Convicted, Prison, Illegal Dispensing

Harold J. Pascal MD, PA – Guilty, Illegal Drug Dispensing; Fraud

Jack I. Dodge MD, SD – License Revoked, Serving 5 years, 92-Count Felony Drug Dealing & Forgery

Kiran Sharma MD, Texas – Prison, $122 million dollar Insurance Theft; Conspiracy, with husband Arun

Arun Sharma MD, Texas – Prison, $122 million dollar Insurance Theft; Conspiracy with wife Kiran

Ramon Scruggs MD, CA – Guilty, Money-laundering

Leyfe R. Anthony MD, Utah – License Revoked, Controlled Substance Violations

Saji Francis MD, NY – Guilty, selling narcotics to teens

James E. Pickens MD, Utah – Prison, Narcotic Distribution

David J. Ciesla MD, Florida – Head of Trauma Center, Tampa, guilty of stealing a bullet in a criminal case

David Gardner MD, CA – Guilty, Money-laundering scheme, Workers' Compensation clinics

William F McArthur MD, Georgia – Prison, Drug Distribution; Conspiracy

Richard Fleming MD, NE – Guilty, Health Care Fraud

Randeep Mann MD, AR – Convicted, Attempted Murder; bombing of another doctor

Khristine Eroshevich MD, L.A. – Guilty, writing prescriptions under false names for Anna Nicole Smith, who died of an overdose

Lawrence Lavin DDS, Philadelphia – Sentenced, 42 years, Cocaine Distribution

Nathaniel Michaels MD, Indiana – Guilty, 'Road Rage' with a handgun

Basil Qandil MD, Detroit – Guilty, illegal sale, 3.7 million narcotic doses

❖

Primum no nocere

As Paramedics we swear to do no harm. But well before we take the Oath we bow to another quite unspoken rule of considerably more gravitas: to overlook the screw-ups and egomaniacal madness of the wayward doctors around us. Yes, early in the career we medics adopt the posture of implausible deniability. Those of us who bother to pay attention are already aware that at least 30% of medications, tests and procedures ordered are unnecessary – many of which will injure and kill the same poor folks we deliver to the hospitals. Ironic, isn't it? Some doctors set about performing all the right procedures – they just do them poorly. Never mind. As a medic you will turn a blind eye toward patient care travesties you see, or risk a short career. It's your choice. Competent physicians navigate the same nerve-wracking path through the same ethical minefield. So do many nurses. And techs. And administrators.

That's the game. Ignore the mania and for God sakes ignore the homicides.

How much proof do you normal people need?

At a medical conference not long ago, accomplished physician-author Marty Makary watched one of his Harvard professors at the podium. The educator looked out at a room of 2,000 physicians and asked, "How many of you know another doctor who should not be practicing because he is too dangerous?"

Every hand went up.

How many bothered to report it?

Not many hands.

What happened above is a fact. And it reveals all we need to know about how thousands of daffy doctors are able to keep right on bungling through their careers, evading appropriate discipline, all the while carving a nasty path of semi-educated carnage. And we in medicine excel at rationalizing untold millions of tragic outcomes because, well, it is after all, the *Twilight Zone*. As long as we are not the patients, it isn't really real. It doesn't really count.

In Makary's revealing book, *Unaccountable,* he describes one Ivy League-trained physician referred to as "Hodad" by his lab coat colleagues, specifically because of this miscreant's ongoing string of patient deaths. "Hodad" is a morose doctor acronym for "hands of death and destruction."

As previously mentioned, Paramedics in our area call them "Double-Ohs." If they happen to be from another country they are conferred the title "TWA's" – Third World Assassins. And America recruits untold thousands, to be turned loose on an unsuspecting public. We just don't tell you who they are.

The fact is, when medics transport you to a hospital we have no way of knowing what kind of care you're in for – whether you are destined to become one of the 680 patients killed today or not. This is no indictment of ER doctors, who are – as far as we can determine – the least problematic of all. Very, very few ER physicians are ever convicted for anything. But they do not keep you in their bailiwick for very long. You get sent off to other doctors, you see. And as long as the code of silence and cloak of secrecy surrounding patient survival and recovery remains the norm, there are precious few ways you can help your own chances.

But you certainly improved your odds when you opened this book. Just absorb the sheer numbers of these characters; their names and the breadth of their sins. And then ask us again how a Paramedic might become a heretic.

❖

James Shin MD, Houston – Guilty, Child Pornography charges

Rogelio Martinez MD, Florida – Guilty, Drug Distribution

David P. Dillon MD, Florida – Guilty, Felony Assault on a Child

Kenneth M. Olds MD, CO

Kelly W. Tucker MD, CO

Pamela W. Pyle MD, SC

Jesse Haggard MD, AR – All found Guilty, Conspiracy, anabolic steroid distribution

Anthony Overton MD, Illinois – Guilty, Sexual Battery on 75-year-old woman

Ethan E. Bickelhaupt MD, KS – Convicted, Illegal Drug use; Drug Distribution

William DeLuca MD, New York

Steven Lynch MD, New York

Douglas Hargrave MD, New York

John Noonan MD, New York

Jeffery Rockmore MD, New York – All guilty, injecting patients with fake Botox at their city of Albany clinic

Paul L. Guidry MD, CA – Guilty, Auto Insurance Fraud

Peter Normann MD, Phoenix – Murder, Manslaughter, patient deaths

Jeremy McCandless MD, Utah – Convicted, Narcotic Distribution

Doyle S. Steele MD, Las Vegas – Guilty, Drug Conspiracy

James M. Stanch MD, NJ – Prison, Narcotic Distribution

Armando Solis MD, Miami – Prison, Narcotics Conspiracy

Keith Sokoloff D.O., Delaware – Guilty, Health Care Fraud

Shirlene Hill MD, AR – Convicted, Substance Abuse

Paul R. Taylor MD, Utah – Pled Guilty, Illegal Drug Distribution

Robert P. Doyle MD, Maine – Reprimand, Inappropriate Sexual Behavior

Mary E. Groves MD, Washington – Denied State License, history of Narcotics use and vehicle accidents

John B. Sireci, D.O., NJ – Pled Guilty, Drug Fraud

James M. Shortt MD, SC – Steroid Distribution Conspiracy

Ernest C. Rose MD, IL – Convicted, Animal Abuse of Horses

Christopher G. Tobin MD, NC – Prison, Illegal Drug Conspiracy

Alexander Theodore MD, Utah – Guilty, Illegal Drug Dispensing

Thomas Tarter MD, ME – License Suspended, failure to maintain proper patient records

Philip G. Wagman MD, PA – Prison, 19 counts, Drug Conspiracy

Donald D. Pope MD, TX – Plead Guilty, Sexual Assault upon 8-year-old girl

Thu Hoa Van MD, MS – Pled Guilty, Illegal Prescriptions

Giles Desmarais PsyD, Las Vegas – Surrendered License, Sex with Patient

Robert Sterling MD, Maine – License Revoked, alcohol use while treating patients

Anthony Galea MD, Canada & U.S. – Tiger Woods physician, Guilty, Drug Smuggling

David G. Evans MD, Las Vegas – Guilty, 15 counts, Sexual Abuse of Minors

❖

Connecticut jury: MD 'guilty' on all 8 counts of patient sexual assault

A superior court jury in Middletown has found Doctor Tory Westbrook guilty of sexually assaulting five women patients while treating them at the *Community Health Center* in Clinton.

Westbrook, age 45 of Glastonbury, faces a maximum 44 years in prison on these convictions alone. And according to prosecutor Peter McShane, the physician still faces 14 more cases.

According to investigators, all of the sexual assaults occurred during a two-year period beginning in 2010.

Westbrook is the husband of Superior Court Judge Dawne Westbrook. He was appointed last year to the Governor's Health Care Cabinet.

❖

Elmer P. Manalo MD, Indiana – License Revoked, Sexual Contact with Patients

Gregory Johns MD, Dothan AL –14-year sentence, Patient Sexual Attacks

Giselle Wildman D.O., Kansas – Surrendered Medical License

Bassam Yassine MD, L.A. – Prison, Illegal Drug Dealing

Warren Williams MD, Baton Rouge – Pled Guilty, Illegal Drug Distribution

Robert Baroody MD, Maine – License Suspended, Sexual Relationship with wife of a patient

Lesley Tripp MD, Maine – License Suspended, Inappropriate Sexual Relationship with patient

James L. Allen MD, Virginia – License Revoked, Child Pornography

David A. Wilbert MD, Phoenix – Conspiracy Steroid Distribution

Larry C. White D.O., Michigan – Pled Guilty, Narcotic Distribution

Sidney Frank MD, Nevada – Reprimand, Gross Negligence

Benjamin M. Brown MD, Maine – License Suspended, Sexual Relationships with staff & patients

Holly Arato MD, Maine – License Suspended, Drug Abuse

Richard T. Gibbs MD, Maine – State Board Reprimand, Treating Patients while under the Influence; Substance Abuse

In Whan Yun MD, Georgia – Fined, Improper Drug Dispensing

Alphonse Yezbick D.O., Michigan – Guilty, Illegal Drug Prescriptions

Renato Mendoza MD, Maine – License Denied, History of Fraud

Randall M. Foster MD, Las Vegas – License Suspension, Failure to Maintain Proper Records of Drug Prescriptions

Andrew Rutland MD, Anaheim – License Surrender, death of yet another abortion patient

Clark Baker MD, Alabama – Pleaded Guilty, Narcotic Trafficking

❖

Do not allow all these convictions impress you. When doctors are released from prison, they get their licenses back. Here is a shameful example:

Physician murders two women; gets his medical license back

A Nashville Tennessee surgeon, who was reissued a medical license after shooting his wife and her mother in 1986, is in trouble again, this time for prescription drug dealing.

Visu Vilvarajah, age 64, served a whopping four years in state prison for the murders, after which time the *Tennessee Board of Medical Examiners* saw no ethical reason to deprive him of the ability to make life and death decisions for unsuspecting patients. Unfortunately his time in prison failed to dampen his penchant for crime: he chose to use his new license to purchase painkillers and become a drug dealer in a lab coat.

In an interview with the *Tennessean News* Vilvarajah stated that just because he killed some people in the past does mean he shouldn't be a doctor.

"I am a talented person. A well-qualified person. I didn't do any crime related to patients. I didn't molest a patient. I am very nice to patients. I only killed my wife because she made me angry."

Had he been a truck driver or a realtor or a chef or a nurse or a contractor, he would have lost his license for life. But we hold physicians to the lowest level of professional discipline in society. Curious, wouldn't you say?

❖

Stephen Pack MD, NY – Prison, stabbed a nurse with a large needle in hospital parking lot

Rodney K. Justin MD, NC – Convicted, Obstruction of Justice & Tax Fraud

Keith Russell, MD, Miami – Sentenced, 8 years, Medicare Fraud

Ronald L. Baird MD, Utah – License Revoked, inappropriate sexual relationships with 5 patients and coworkers

Lawrence Simons MD, Kansas – Guilty, "pill mill" case after 59 patients died

Jock Simon MD, NJ – New convictions for troubled doctor

Esther Wadley, MD, MO – Guilty, Conspiracy to Murder ex-husband

Raymond Adamcik MD, FL – Guilty, Disorderly Conduct, "Captain America burrito-in-pants groping" case

Mark B. Kabins MD, Las Vegas – Guilty, Falsification of Medical Charts

Dale Pearlman MD, CA – Ethics Review following "head lice treatment scam"

James Shin MD, Fort Worth – Convicted, Child Porn, former chief of medicine, *John Peter Smith Hospital*

James M. Bachstein MD, Tenn. – Probation, Inappropriate Prescribing of Narcotics

James H. Ellegood MD, St. Louis – Medicare Fraud Home Health scam

Robert W. Osteen MD, Tenn. – Probation, Diverted Medication for personal use

Larry G. Andrew MD, Utah – Convicted, 8 Counts, Sexual Battery on a Patient

Stephen L. Seldon MD, Las Vegas – Prison, Fake Botox Injection clinic

Ronald Poulin MD, Virginia – Prison, 28 Counts Insurance Fraud

❖

New York doctor gets jail; argues that her "other personality" sold drugs

An MD who claimed one of her 'alternate personalities' was to blame for her role in a prescription-drug ring was sentenced to three years in prison.

To the shock of her lawyer, Doctor Diana Williamson, age 56, received a prison term and was ordered by Manhattan Federal Court Judge Loretta Preska to be taken into custody immediately.

The judge also fined the errant doctor and ordered her to repay $300,000 in restitution. Williamson pleaded guilty to Conspiracy and Health Care fraud.

❖

Ann Campbell MD, Alabama – Prison, 5-year term, Drug Study Falsification, faking patient charts

Thomas Lover D.C., Ohio – Prison, Worker's Compensation Fraud

Ramon Scruggs MD, Sacramento – Convicted, Illegal Drugs to Athletes

George L. Aycock MD, SC – Guilty, Illegal Drug Dispensing

Christopher G. Wayne MD Miami Beach – 6 years, $1.6M Medicare Theft

Eugene P. O'Donnell MD, L.A. – Convicted, Tax Evasion

Walter G. Broadnax MD, Ohio – Medical Coding Fraud

Elizabeth Robertson MD, N.C. – Guilty, Obtaining Narcotics by Fraud

Stephen P. Wolf MD, Oklahoma – Mental Institution, stabbing 9-year-old son to death

Bradley E. Baker MD, Oregon – State Order of Emergency Medical License Suspension, Substance Abuse

Callie H. Harpin MD, Houston – Prison, $30M Wheelchair Prescription Fraud

Michel Chait MD, New York – Guilty, Narcotic Distribution

Robert Cleveland MD, Shreveport – Guilty, Wheelchair Prescription Fraud

Ira Klein MD, Houston – Prison, 11 years, Fraud; Conspiracy to Murder a U.S. Prosecutor

Kevin A. Lang MD, Wisconsin – 5-year term, Sexual Assault, 5 female patients under sedation

Jerome Lentini MD, Portland – Convicted, Fake Botox Scam

Franklin Sutherland MD, VA – Guilty, Illegal Narcotic Sales

Linda S. Cheek MD, VA – Convicted, Medicare Fraud

Vu Le MD, Orange County, CA – Sentenced, 4 years, Drug-running

Howard Berkowitz MD, Atlanta – Guilty, Health Care Fraud

Arthur Hargraves MD, Atlanta – Sentenced, 3 years, Fraud

William W. Hampton MD, L.A. – Convicted, $9M dollar "Sweaty Palm Surgery" scam

❖

Ohio MD gets sentence reduction after assaulting dozens of women

A Cleveland Ohio gynecologist in prison for sexually assaulting at least 30 of his patients, has been issued a drastically reduced sentence. He will now serve a fraction of the time in prison of which he was initially scheduled.

Doctor Assam Ahmed, found guilty in 2004, was originally ordered to serve a term of 45 years in Ohio State Prison. Ahmed's attorneys filed for a re-sentencing in 2006 and his sentence has now been reduced to 11 years.

As a result, Ahmed will be released in 2015.

❖

Hung T. Nguyen MD, NY – Guilty, Illegal Dispensing Narcotics

Randy S. Lentz MD, Florida – Guilty, Conspiracy to Commit Fraud

Torrino Jennings MD, VA – Convicted, 1,000,000 Illegal Drug Transactions

Mamdouk Bahna MD, L.A. – Guilty, Health Care Fraud

Daniel Puffenberger MD, NY – Guilty, Medicare Fraud

Thomas Wilkins MD, PA – Guilty, Illegal Drug Prescriptions

Phillip Wagman MD, NJ – Sentenced, 19 years, Fraud

Roberto Rodriguez MD, Miami – Guilty, HIV Infusion Fraud

Carlos Garrido MD, Miami – Guilty, HIV Infusion Fraud

Carmen Del Cueto MD, Miami – Guilty, HIV Infusion Fraud

Kurien C. Abraham MD, NC – Convicted, Repeated DUI crashes

Peter S. Grigg MD, Denver – Convicted, selling drug prescriptions in Walmart parking lot

Ali Salim MD, Ohio – 36-year term; Rape, Murder, 'doing inhumane things' to woman's corpse

Phillip Riback MD, NY – Guilty, Sexual Abuse, young boys

Louis Cannella, Jr. MD, Wisconsin – Sentenced, 4 years, Illegal Narcotic Sales

Michael Millette MD, Iowa – Convicted, selling 62 million doses of narcotics

Mark Campano MD, Ohio – Convicted, Illegal Possession of Explosives after blowing himself up

Charles Cowden MD, Tenn. – Indicted, Rape, Medical Fraud

Delvin Littell MD, Knoxville – Guilty, Narcotic Drug-running

Loren Nichols MD, Tenn. – Parole Hearing, Illegal Narcotic Dispensing

Horace Bledsoe MD, Lexington KY – Pled Guilty, Drug Diversion, Medical Records Falsification

Roger Brown MD, Florida – Convicted, Drug Ring Scheme

Kathleen Hagen MD, New Jersey – Prison Release Program, following the murder of her parents

Jeffery Friedlander MD, Tampa – Convicted, Drug Scheme, Medicare Fraud

Darryl C. Harris MD, Beaumont, TX – Guilty, Medical Testing Fraud

John M. Felton MD, Boston – Guilty, intent to have sex with a 6-year-old boy

Jorge A. Martinez MD, Ohio – Life-term, Fraud; Narcotics Distribution resulting in patient death

Frederic Feit MD, Manalapan NJ – Prison, Health Care Fraud

Doyle S. Steele MD, Las Vegas – Prison, 'Drugs for Sex' case

Mel Levine, MD, North Carolina – Suicide prior to Child Sexual Abuse trial

Josyann Abisaab MD, NY – License Suspended, Failure to Report Gunshot Wound, NFL player Plaxico Burress

Brian Shaffer MD, NJ

Giacomo Mangiaracina MD, NJ

Louis Tsarouhas MD, NJ – All Guilty, Tax Evasion; Kickbacks

Oliver W. Herndon MD, PA – 11-year term, Narcotics Distribution

Jeffrey Dardinger MD, KY – Guilty, secretly filming nude girl

❖

His name was Jefferson Moore and he was a marvelous physical specimen. He was six feet, seven inches tall and weighed 248 pounds. The man should have had a red "S" on his chest. If you are thinking that he sounds like a pro football player you'd be half-right. Because the sad truth is on this afternoon he'd just been released by the San Diego Chargers and today was the last day of his life.

The pre-season games had come and gone and the Chargers – like every other team in the NFL – were forced to make the painful decision of telling two dozen world-class athletes that they weren't quite good enough. One of those players was Jefferson Moore, an offensive lineman, and he took the news worse than most. He cleaned out his locker, packed his bags and headed out through Mission Valley toward the 805 freeway. And somewhere along his trip he decided to start playing with a pistol in his hand, aiming it at his head, pointing it at cars nearby, waving it at the sky. This went on for about 10 minutes, when someone called 911 to report Moore's very strange behavior. No one knew who he was, of course. As fate would have it, an off-duty sheriff's deputy happened to be traveling that same freeway, and found himself several cars behind Moore's, near enough to see the weapon in his hand as he held it aimlessly out the window. The officer followed him all the way home and pulled up behind him in an underground parking area. With both cars stopped the cop ordered Moore to put the weapon down. Instead, in what for all the world resembled a 'suicide by cop' maneuver, Moore advanced on the officer and pointed his gun without firing. The deputy shot Moore in the chest four times.

EMS archives for that day report that it took us five minutes to get there, Dave and I, working on a hospital-based medic team called *Lifesaver 1.* We found Moore lying on his back on the concrete floor, surrounded by a half-dozen police officers. We got quickly to work – ripping open the shirt; assessing the bullet wounds; applying oxygen; double IV lines of Lactated Ringers. Unlike the movies, there is rarely much bleeding in a gunshot wound, and there was very little here. We were impressed with the quality of his heart and lung sounds. Moore writhed on the ground, slipping in and out of consciousness. We got the big man onto a backboard, then to the gurney with some difficulty, and had him at the closest ER within minutes.

At the hospital the trauma team leaped into action, and all proceeded normal for a time. As was typical with the Lifesaver protocols, Dave and I functioned as part of the trauma team – which is just one reason why hospital-based medics are more competent than most. A stat chest x-ray revealed that Moore's heart was intact and although his lungs had been penetrated, they were functioning far better than you'd think. The guess was that several of the shots had simply not gone through the muscular chest wall. Amazing. We had two physicians working the case now, and neither of them appeared eager to take the next logical step. Moore was alive after being shot in the chest four times. He was conscious enough to writhe and move his arms and his vital signs were better than they should have been. The man needed his chest opened and he needed it now. Dave and I looked at each other more than once during that hour, wondering why in hell these two MDs thought it was more important to stand at the x-ray glass admiring his lung function, than simply opening his chest, or getting him up to surgery for someone more qualified.

But there they stood, gaping at the x-rays. Wow. Look at those lungs. Tick-tock, tick-tock. Had we taken him to a trauma center twenty minutes further, Moore's surgery would be half-over by now. But what the football player got instead were two physician bystanders admiring his body. They just couldn't seem to stem their veneration long enough to play real doctor. They were all caught up in lamentable awe that Jefferson Moore could still be alive.

Fifty-eight minutes later, he wasn't.

❖

Larry E. Perry MD, Tenn. – License Suspended, Patient Sexual Misconduct

Rexford Agbenohevi MD, Tenn. – License Suspended, Inappropriate Sexual Relationship, with a patient in medical exam rooms

Paul Emerson MD, Detroit – Guilty, Prescription Resulting in Death; Illegal Prescribing Narcotics

Arie Van Der Wiede MD, Michigan – Prison, Criminal sexual relations with child under 13

Brant G. Kersey MD, Tenn. – License Reprimand, Repeated Prescribing Errors

James H. Pogue MD, Tenn. – License Reprimand, Unprofessional, Unethical, Dishonest Conduct

David C. Winkler MD, San Antonio – Convicted, Child Pornography Case

Sylvain Junger MD, Passaic NJ – Convicted, Patient Sexual Molestation

Daniel Healy MD, Arcadia, CA – Convicted, "Pain Killers for Cash"

Robert C. Vonborstel MD, Oregon –Surrendered Medical License, Illegally prescribing narcotics; sexual relationship with drug-addicted patient

❖

Diabolic doctor-duo and their 'little house of horrors'

In a case that is cringeworthy even here in bizarre world, two Hamilton Ohio physicians have been tried and sent to prison for their decades of sexually assaulting children.

Investigators were able to prove that brothers Scott and Mark Blankenberg, 56-year old twin pediatricians, had been molesting young male patients for at least 20 years.

Doctor Scott Blankenberg admitted guilt to eight felony counts and was sentenced to 13 years in Ohio state prison. The eight charges included; Compelling Prostitution; Pandering sexually-oriented material of children; Illegal use of Minors and nudity material; Unlawful Sexual Conduct with children.

Doctor Mark Blankenberg will serve 21 years in prison for nearly identical crimes.

Identical twins. Identical specialties. Identical atrocities in smallville, USA, allowed to continue for two decades. Why? Well, because at least four other pediatricians aware of this outrage remained resolutely silent.

And we turn our patients over to these people.

❖

Peter LaFuria MD, Louisiana – Guilty, 20 counts, Patient Sexual Assault; Filming nude patients

Jack L. Glisson MD, Tenn. – Probation, performed surgery without a license

Douglas W. Kane MD, Tenn. – Probation, treating patients while under the influence

Pravin Vasoya MD, NJ – Guilty, Intent to Sell Narcotics

Gregory Johns MD, Alabama – Guilty, Sexually Abusing 2 Patients

Daryn W. Peterson MD, Las Vegas – Convicted, Health Care Fraud

Phillip A. Knorr MD, Santa Cruz, CA –Reprimand, Probation, Incomplete Care of Patient, Negligence

Harry A. Zain MD, Tenn. – Guilty of Assault

John R. Wickerman MD, Tenn. – License Suspended, Inappropriate Sexual Contact with a Patient

Carmen Por MD, Ohio – Guilty, Theft, Cash & Credit Card from patients & staff

John T. Tiano MD, SC – Guilty, Conspiracy, Health Fraud

Alexander Chernowitz MD, Tenn. – License Restricted, Substance Abuse

George Koral MD, California – Released from Prison, Maintain License Revocation, Attempted Murder of Wife by Arson

Putnam Breed MD, Mass – Convicted, Cremation Fraud

Fabian Aurignac MD, LA – Guilty, Fraud

Yaseed Essa MD, Ohio – Life term, Murder, his wife by cyanide

Sukhdarshan Bedi MD, Illinois – Guilty, Drug Scheme, Obstruction of Justice

Emenike U. John MD – License Revoked, Multiple Sexual Assaults of a patient

Pravin Vasoya MD, NJ – Guilty, Intent to Sell Narcotics

John H. Story MD, Wyoming – 15-year sentence, Multiple Patient Rape

Tony Shiu MD, CA - Prison, Patient Rape; photos of nude patients

❖

Maryland surgeons found guilty in heart stent scam

Another Baltimore heart surgeon has been convicted of numerous criminal acts which, among other felonies, included the implanting of unnecessary cardiac stents into at least 200 patients. He then stole hundreds of thousands of dollars from insurers, billing for procedures that ought never have been done.

Doctor John R. McLean, age 59, was sentenced to eight years in prison, according to the Maryland U.S. Attorney's Office.

Nicholas DiGiulio, a special agent in charge for the *U.S. Department of Health and Human Services*, said, "Placing unnecessary stents in the hearts of patients is a crime of unthinkable proportions. We will continue to bring justice to those physicians who practice greed, rather than medicine."

McLean is one of at least five surgeons to be convicted for fraudulent stent operations in recent years, including a Louisiana MD who was sentenced to a 10-year term in 2009. Another Maryland cardiologist, Mark G. Midei, had his medical license revoked on similar allegations and was found guilty of Medical Malpractice last October. He faces at least 45 more lawsuits by patients.

Studies have consistently proven that heart vessel stents, which prop open narrow arteries to improve blood flow, are overused. A *Journal of the American Medical Association* review in 2011 found that at least 50% of stent procedures in one treatment category are questionable or outright wrong. Yet the surgical shickery goes on unabated.

Both McLean and Midei were found to have purposely exaggerated the degree of arterial blockage in their patients and falsified medical records to justify the stents, which are inserted via a relatively simple procedure that typically costs $10,000-$20,000. McLean was criminally indicted for crimes committed between 2003-2007, while employed by *Peninsula Regional Medical Center* in Salisbury. Midei wreaked his havoc at *St. Joseph Hospital* in Baltimore.

❖

Jose Bolanos MD, San Jose – Guilty, Patient Sexual Assault

Sohrab Shafinia D.O., MI – Guilty, Narcotics Conspiracy

Jaroslav P. Stulc MD, Maine – Guilty, Fraud, Sexual Misconduct

Parvis K Berjis MD, LA – Prison, Workers' Comp/Auto Insurance Fraud

Masood Bamdad MD, CA – Convicted, 13 counts Drug-dealing

Pradeep Svrivastava MD, MD – Guilty, $16M Tax Evasion

Manual Barbiete MD, Florida – HIV Infusion Fraud

Godfrey Mbonu MD, NY – Sentenced, Medicare Fraud

Irfan Nawaz MD, Florida – Guilty, Internet Child Sexual Exploitation

Manoj Motwani, MD, CA – Convicted, Battery, girlfriend while driving

James Rice MD, San Diego – Guilty, Prescription Forgery

Mazoltuy Borukhova MD, NY – Convicted, Murder Conspiracy

Mohammed F. Salek MD, Nevada – Convicted, Health Care Fraud

Rajitha Goli MD, St. Louis – Medicare Fraud; Home Health Care

William H. Ayres MD, San Francisco – Guilty, 8 counts, Child Molestation

Medhut Shenouda MD, NY – 12-year term, Attempted Murder of his wife by injecting insulin

Suresh Shah MD, Palm Springs – Guilty, Sexual Harassment

Byron Glenn MD, Illinois – Convicted, passing fake money order

Narendra K. Agrawal, MD Ohio – 3-year sentence, Drug Trafficking

Walter Proano MD, Miami – Guilty, Health Care Fraud

Hung T. Nguyen MD, NY – Guilty, Illegal Dispensing, Narcotics

Rogelio Naranja MD, Maine – Probation, Unprofessional Conduct

Vu Le MD, Orange County CA – Sentenced 4 years, Drug-running

Akiva Abraham MD, Albany NY – Guilty, Arson; Insurance Fraud

Augusto Loaiza MD, Florida – Ordered to Surrender License

Mehendra Udani MD, L.A. – Prison, multiple Patient Molestation convictions

Michael A. Taylor MD, Mass. – Medicaid Fraud; Illegal Drug-dealing

Suresh Hemrajani MD, New York – Convicted, $700,000 HIV Med Fraud

Rakesh Anand MD, Indiana – Guilty, Amphetamine Drug Dealing

Dr. Alphonso Berry MD, Detroit – Guilty, $13M Psychotherapy Fraud

Felix Lanting MD, Staten Island – Convicted, Drug-dealing from home

Meera Sachdeva MD, MS – Guilty, $8M Cancer Cure Fraud

Mark Weinberger MD, Indiana – Convicted, Health Care Fraud

Cary Stephen Feldman D.O., SD – Guilty, Grand Theft by Deception

Carl G. Koplin MD, Conn – Guilty, Child Pornography

David Wexler MD, Manhattan – 20-year term, Narcotic Distribution

Soraya Abbassian MD, Portland – Guilty, Criminally Negligent Homicide, death of a patient

Steven Hall MD, Kentucky – Manslaughter, ran over his wife with a party boat

Melvin Morse MD, Delaware – Guilty of 'waterboard' torturing his daughter

❖

Doctor Earl Bradley: "Worst child predator in U.S. history"

A Delaware physician will spend the rest of his life in prison for sexually abusing dozens of children over more than a decade, according to Superior Court Judge William Carpenter.

Doctor Earl Bradley, age 58, was sentenced to 14 life terms for 14 counts of first-degree rape. Bradley was also sentenced to 160 years for numerous other counts of assault and sexual exploitation.

This particular deviant was initially charged on 471 counts of rape and molestation of 103 child patients – 102 girls and one boy.

"You will never be in a position to harm a child again," Judge Carpenter told Bradley. He added that the serial pedophile had violated the trust of his patients and their families. "You have severely violated that trust, and you have shamed your profession. You appear to be the worst child predator in U.S. history."

Prosecutor Paula Ryan stated, "Earl Bradley committed unspeakable acts upon those who could not speak for themselves. To make indescribable and horrific matters even worse, he videotaped these incidents for his own perverse pleasure, endlessly editing and copying, permanently memorializing his attacks on these children for his own twisted collection."

Because MDs rarely report the monsters in their midst, Bradley escaped prosecution for two decades, while more and more children – some as young as three months – were victimized. After his arrest investigators discovered that the *Delaware State Medical Board*; *Beebe Medical Center*; the *Delaware Department of Justice*, and **other pediatricians**, were all in violation of the law, by not reporting what they knew about Bradley's outrageous mistreatment of children.

❖

Amar Nath Bhandry MD, Ok City – Guilty, Health Care Fraud

Nolan D. Crisp MD, Missouri – Guilty, Drug-dealing in parking lots

Robert Lilly MD, NC – Guilty, Sexual Assault, 73-year old patient

Kenneth Seen MD, NC – Guilty, Patient Assault, stuck his tongue into a patient's mouth and had it bitten off

Mikhail Presman MD, NY - Guilty, $2.8M Health Care Fraud

Robert Ignasiak MD, Florida – Convicted, Drug-running; Medical Fraud

Briana Boyd MD, Kentucky – 6-year term, drunk-driving crash

Linda Cheek MD, Virginia – Guilty, 172 counts, Narcotics Distribution

David C. Miller MD, MN – Guilty, Narcotics Theft

Donald Gibson MD, Texas – Convicted, Health Care Fraud

Leonard Stambler MD, NY – Convicted, Narcotics Drug-running

Jasubhai Desai MD, Detroit – Guilty, Murder, former girlfriend

Diane Shafer MD, WV – Guilty, Operating a "Pill Mill"

Daniel G. Walters MD, CA – Guilty, Sexual Battery, 18-year old intern

John Maye OB/GYN, NY – Convicted, 33 counts, Drug-dealing

Leonard Joachim MD, NJ – Guilty, Patient Sexual Assault

Barry DeRan MD, Ohio – Sentenced, 28 months, Drug-dealing

Houshang Pavehzadeh DC, L.A. – Guilty, $1M Insurance Theft

David Nash MD, Alabama – Convicted, Murder for Hire

Edgar Lockett MD, Amarillo – Convicted, $1.4M Tax Evasion

Gustave Drivas MD, NY – Guilty, $77M Insurance Fraud

Robert Gibbs MD, NY – Convicted, Narcotics Trafficking

Van E. Scott MD, Penn – Guilty, 10 counts, Illegal Prescriptions

Charles M. Howe MD, Tenn. – Guilty, 14 counts, Drug-dealing

Richard R. Ruth MD, Penn – Convicted, Drug-dealing

John Ott MD, Wash. DC – 20-years, Sexual Assaults, 14 children

Fernando G. Ramos MD, Utah – Guilty, Drug-dealing

Larry A. Hearne MD, SC – Convicted, Tax Evasion

Kathleen Lake MD, Illinois – Guilty, Drug Fraud

John Green MD, Maryland – Guilty, diagnostic testing kickbacks

Robert Dicky MD, Wash DC – Convicted, Child Pornography

Paul Ostergaard MD, NJ – Guilty, bribes for testing scheme

Samir Zaky MD, CT – Convicted, 28 counts, Medicare Theft

Curtis Holden MD, Washington – Guilty, 32 counts, Insurance Theft

Daniel H. Jebans MD, SC – Guilty, Drug-dealing conspiracy

Bruce M. Becker MD, RI – Convicted, buying alcohol for teenagers

Fitzgerald A. Hudson MD, MI – Guilty, Health Care Fraud

Gwendolyn Washington MD, MI – 10-year term, Drug Trafficking, Fraud

Eugene Goldman MD, Penn – Guilty, kickback scheme

Randy Spicer D.O., Arizona – 13-year term, sex with a child

Margaret Edwards MD, Ohio – Convicted, child starvation case

Scott D. Anderson MD, CA – Guilty, Patient Sexual Abuse

Zakaria Oweiss MD, Wash DC – Prison, Murder of wife with a hammer

Michael Mastromarino MD, NY – Convicted, Selling Human Body Parts

Kenneth B. Woods MD, L.A. – Convicted, oral sex on a 9-year old girl

Arnold P. Weiss MD, Rhode Island – Guilty, stolen coin scam

Karl Long MD, Penn – Guilty, Wife Murder, suffocation

William Lagrada MD, Edison NJ – Guilty, Diagnostic Tests scam

Ovid Mercene MD, Los Angeles – Guilty, Medicare Theft, homeless patients

Cleveland J. Enmon Jr., Florida – Convicted, 90 counts, Drug-dealing

Dennis Wicks MD, Rapid City Iowa – Convicted, Tax Evasion

Mohamed Kadirsahib MD, Canada – Convicted, Patient Sexual Assault

David T. Montaldi, Intern, Michigan – 32-year sentence, Infant Rape

Lana Le Chabrier MD, Sacramento – 6-year prison term, Insurance Fraud

Ashok Bararia MD, New Jersey – Guilty, MRI kickback scheme

Michael C. Lam MD, New Jersey – Guilty, Illegal Drug Distribution

Eliseo Roquiz MD, Penn – Convicted, Income Tax Evasion

Hoshang Pormir MD, California – Guilty, Illegal patient drugging case

Tahir Usman Mir, MD, Indiana – Confession, Drugs-for-Sex case

Joon Chong MD, Cincinnati – Guilty, Prescription Drug-dealing

Mahmoud Y. Hindi MD, Kentucky – Suicide in jail; shot two men during a homeowners' association meeting

Michael P. Stein MD, New Jersey – Guilty, $725,000 Blue Cross Fraud

Adam W. Lebowitz MD, Atlanta – Guilty, Child Sex Enticement

Paul A. Taylor MD, Salt Lake City – Illegal Narcotic Distribution

Mark Felton MD, Boston MA – Guilty, attempted sexual encounter with a 6-year-old boy

Beau Boshers MD, Palm Beach – Guilty, Money-laundering

Vinay Bararia MD, Las Vegas – Guilty, Drug-dealing in Centennial Hills Hospital parking lot

David V. Gierlus MD, Iowa – 8-year sentence, traded drugs for sex with 18 female patients

Adam Levinson MD, New York – Guilty, secret camera, filming up women's skirts on the subway

Fort Hood mass murder-doctor left years of warning signs

Army physician Nidal Hasan, sentenced to death for shooting 45 soldiers in 2009 on a Texas military base, was known as "a ticking time bomb" to those who knew him years before the massacre.

The 43 year-old psychiatrist, who held the rank of major at the time of his outrage, made repeated assertions that Muslims were being persecuted by the United States. While lecturing at the *Uniformed Services University Health Sciences* in Bethesda, Maryland, Hasan would tell students that "Shari 'a law transcends the Constitution of the United States." He also told students that "homicidal bombers are rewarded for their acts with 72 virgins in heaven."

In fact, even before Hasan achieved a Master's Degree in Public Health, he was considered by physician staff and students alike to be a total misfit for the program. Court records show that he had serious discipline problems and did not relate well at all with psychiatric patients. Upon graduation from the Pentagon medical school, his business card included the initials "SOA" which is common to jihadist websites. It stands for "soldiers of Allah."

According to one classmate, "He would stand there in uniform pledging allegiance to the Koran."

The murder of 13 soldiers at Fort Hood – and the wounding of 32 – was enough of a tragedy for any society. Perhaps worse than the bloodshed is the undeniable fact that Hasan's medical colleagues and superiors refused to act on what they knew about this maniac. We submit they bear a significant level of responsibility for the murders as well.

But then, when it comes to hiding dragons, that happens to be one area in which health care professionals consistently excel.

Hasan joins 147 other physicians sent to death row nationwide.

❖

Giocondo Navek MD, Fort Bragg NC – Murder-Suicide, girlfriend

Jose Katz MD, Closter NJ – Guilty, 19M Patient Care Fraud

William Holmes MD, Turin Italy – Convicted, Murder of his wife

Lewis Jackson MD, Wash DC – Guilty, Patient Sexual Assault

George Doodnaught MD, Toronto – Guilty, 21 Patient Sexual Assaults

Timothy G. Roses MD, Iowa – Guilty, Murder-Suicide, girlfriend

Michael Mockovak MD, Seattle – 20-year term, Conspiracy to Murder

Kevin P. Anderson MD, L.A. – Guilty, Murder, doctor-girlfriend

Frederick Field MD, Oregon – Convicted, sexually assaulting patients under sedation

Boris Sachakov MD, Brooklyn – Convicted, Fraud, billing insurance companies for non-existent patients and procedures

Norman Barwin MD, Ontario Canada – Guilty, Artificial Insemination Incompetency

Charles Nguyen MD, Ohio – 30 years, Rape, Kidnapping

Marjan Jafari MD, Newark, NJ – Guilty, Kickbacks, Conspiracy

William Ellien MD, Savannah GA –Convicted, Sex for Drugs case

Steven Rios DC, Philadelphia – 4 years, Auto Insurance Fraud

George Matthews MD, Maryland – Convicted, Drug-dealing

Scott Houghton MD, Madison CT – Guilty, Drug-dealing

Viwath Bhuthimethee MD, St. Louis – Guilty, Felony Drug-running

David H. Scanlan MD, Penn – Convicted, Child Porn Distribution

Paul K. Holden MD, Phoenix – Convicted, Drug Theft

Donald Quinn DDS, Detroit – Convicted, Patient Sexual Assault

Adelina Herrero, MD, Michigan – Guilty, $1.3M Medicare Theft

Joshua D. Baron MD, Chicago – Guilty, Drugs for Sex case

❖

The case of the tail wagging the doc

So perhaps by now you suspect that when it comes to clinical cretinism you have heard it all. No you haven't.

Sit back and appreciate this unexaggerated beauty:

Last July *Los Angeles County Sheriff* detectives raided an urgent care clinic in the city of Glendora. After a two-month investigation they were convinced the clinic's drug prescription patterns were, well, just a bit askew.

The good news one day was that Doctor Rolando L. Atiga was able to interpret the x-ray one of his patients had brought along, well enough to prescribe pretty much any narcotic painkiller she wanted. He could tell by the x-ray she was honestly in agony.

"Do you want to try some Vicoden?" he asked. "Roxicodone? Maybe Valium? Xanex?" He was really quite accommodating. He even pointed out a hip bone as the probable cause of her suffering.

Of course the bad news was that the patient was an undercover cop and the x-ray was the skeletal image of her German

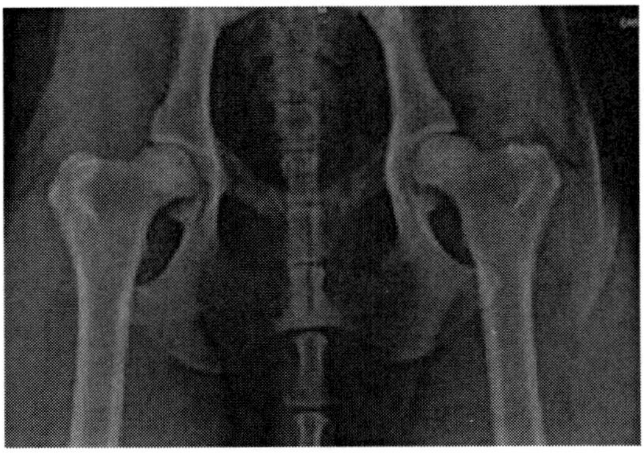

shepherd. Kindly note the tail:

So just between us, which aspect of health care makes you feel better? That your personal physician might lie to you; falsify patient records and push drugs? Or that he might be incompetent enough to actually think this is an x-ray of a human being?

Alas, Doctor Rolando L. Atiga was escorted from his urgent care clinic in handcuffs. He was charged with multiple counts of felony prescription fraud. Do you care to know what the good doctor said to the police as they tucked him carefully into the backseat of a patrol car?

"I don't know if I did something wrong or something right."

We don't call it the *Twilight Zone* for nothing.

❖

And finally, we suspect our society would suffer considerably less lab coat lunacy, if we simply mimicked Saudi Arabia for a decade or two:

Saudi doctor to be whipped for molesting patient

In the eastern province of Ihsa a Saudi Arabian court has ordered a senior physician to be lashed 120 times as the result of his patient molestation conviction.

Under Saudi law the doctor's name is not publicized, but according to health minister Abdullah Al Rabeeah, the physician was a consultant at a large hospital in the province of Ihsa when he was taken into custody. He was found guilty of sexually molesting at least one woman and of repeated hospital rule violations which required him to have a female nurse present when examining female patients.

The MD was also sentenced to 18 months in prison.

Immutable Law #9

No profession in society generates more crime; injures and kills more people; nor evades more appropriate discipline, than physicians. Yet our job is to turn you over to them and never tell you which ones are likely to harm you. So we don't.

"Men occasionally stumble over the truth. But most pick themselves up and hurry off as if nothing has happened."

—Sir Winston Churchill

Chapter Ten

It ought to be a soul-cleansing experience.
But it is instead quite paralyzing to realize the
focus of your life's work is inherently illogical

A world movement was born the day former Vice President Al Gore revealed his global warming documentary, "*An Inconvenient Truth*." Now whether you happen to believe that the human race contributes to earth climate change or not, we submit our own exasperating truth – one that can be openly appreciated by conservatives and liberals alike:

Rescuers save an awful lot of imbeciles.

Yes, for decades my colleagues and I have retrieved the wretched lives of more cretins than we can count. And every day, as certain as sunrise, some mighty fine men and women across this nation get the call; hop into their bright-hued Tonka Toys; flip on the bells and whistles and dash out to salvage a hundred more. Some will lose their own lives trying. You'd think we'd learn.

Once, in 3:00 a.m. loon-laden stupor, I sat slumped in an ambulance seat too tired to sleep, and actually scribbled this onto a medical chart:

"Churls and creeps, stinkers and slime. Lowlifes, vulgarians, birdbrains and swine. Snots and scoundrels, racists and stupes. Gangsters, clodpolls, golems and dupes.

We save them.

Nutjobs and morons, dingbats and nitwits. Pinheads, lamebrains, dipsticks and halfwits.

We save them.

Varlet, rapscallion, barbarian and all? Thug and fiend and Neanderthal? Assassin or dumbass, bomber or rook? Villain or terrorist, gunman or crook?

We save them."

Why?

The history of ethical theory tells us there is more than one way to think about this pesky little matter of ratbag rescue. It was 250 years ago, for example, when Immanuel Kant proffered his brilliant thoughts on right and wrong. What we now call Kantian Ethics carries impressive weight in our classrooms and courtrooms, even today. Kant's Principle of Humanity argued that people should be treated humanely by saving their lives and alleviating suffering – proper respect for personhood. And that is indeed the fundamental principle of EMS response, no question. Of course, it was also Kant who proposed that moral expectations are based on what he called the Categorical Imperative. Unethical behavior, he said, violates this societal imperative and is therefore not rational. Alas, we expend enormous resources rescuing the 'irrational' everyday of the year. The question of today is, how rational is that?

❖

"All things are subject to interpretation. Whichever interpretation prevails at a given time is a function of power – not truth."

Friedrich Nietzsche

❖

Previous thinkers like Thomas Hobbes and John Locke had also argued that moral requirements are based on standards of rationality; that those of equal worth are deserving of equal respect. One might logically deduce from this, we submit, that those of unequal worth are 'deserving' of a lesser degree of respect. And we submit further that some are not deserving of the lives and limbs of rescuers, who in current day rationale are socially obligated to save the demented from themselves.

Bernard Gert grew famous in part because he expounded that there are no true ethical rules of good will at all – only ethical ideals. Our obligations in a moral society, he surmised, are defined by shunning injury and acts of bad will. Gert's opinion was that we share no obligation to promote good – but rather to minimize the causes of evil. Those of rational mind would treat all persons with the aim of non-injury. Gert argued that *causing harm* is immoral, but *requiring citizens to help other persons*, which includes acting to prevent harm they themselves create, is also wrong.

Over the extent of recorded human history plenty has been written – and much wisdom can be mined – from the cogency of those of considerably brighter mind than our own. From Confucius to Aristotle, from Descartes to Socrates, dozens of intellectuals have proffered enlightened points of view on the matter of exactly how an ethical society ought to behave.

Yet as varied as their observations have been; as different as their backgrounds were, these philosophic giants have a single, irrefutable weakness in common: not one of them lives in the 21st century. The population of the United States during Kant's lifetime was an estimated 5,000,000. Today it is 317,000,000. The result of such meteoric township bloating is a stunning volume of despicable behavior. During the British Elizabethan era of Thomas Hobbes, for example, felons were so severely punished that they were often pressed to death in public by placing increasingly heavy weights on their chests until they suffocated. Nietzsche's experience in Germany included public hangings by chains for looting, armed robbery and rape. Neither Hume nor Hegel nor Spinoza nor Thomas Aquinas was ever forced to consider atrocities that even our own third-graders must grapple with today:

- Drive-by murders and legal pharmaceutical poisoning of the masses
- The daily homicides of strangers in violent cities
- Secret cameras in doctors' offices
- School shootings and unnecessary surgeries for profit
- The bombing of innocents out of political scorn
- Road rage, drugs running rampant and airliners blown from the sky

Who else has noticed that when it comes to the acceptance of depravity in any society, on some cosmic clock we may not yet readily grasp – the pendulum swings? And we strongly suspect that America's tolerance pendulum will commence its painfully slow, inevitable arc back toward the cold hard intolerance of outrageous behavior, as seen in our past. And when that day arrives – when we have stomached quite enough dead children in schools and enough nearly dead fools on highways – we fully anticipate that heads will nod in agreement with John Stuart Mill's clarifications of Jeremy Bentham's Utilitarianism. This belief touts that the moral worth of any action is determined by its resulting outcome. Injured fools need not apply. Future debates will surely rage on just how much lifesaving ought to be extended to those who demonstrate the temerity to actually assault rescuers who risk their own lives saving them. Mill, who expanded much of his inductive logic from Avicenna, ancient Persia's finest physician/philosopher, argued that moral thinkers had scribed a litany of unconvincing and unimpressive theories that could be better whittled into a single standard of ethics – one that allows society to more readily determine what is right and what is wrong. He proffered the Principle of Utility – the "greatest happiness" theorem – as the basic foundation of ethical behavior. *Conduct is moral in proportion to its provision of happiness for everybody else.* Misbehaviors are immoral if they produce less happiness among the rest of us. This offers up an uncomplicated proposition for rescue, although admittedly a sobering one. A dispassionate assessment of utilitarian rescue protocol might support acts of lifesaving which contribute to overall wellbeing and reduced suffering. Yet in a more critical future – a time when a rescue might involve extreme danger to the rescuer, or continued peril to society by prolonging the life of, say, a career rapist shot by police, or the habitually careless on the streets – we just might no longer extend the privilege of life-saving at all.

Mill's utilitarian advocates believe that conduct is right – graded on the curve of other possible conduct – if it leads to the optimal balance of societal tranquility. Conversely, an action is wrong to the extent that it results in societal distress. The observation from here is that – in our all-out attempt to save scoundrels as saints – we do enormous injustice to the wellbeing of the community. Mill refined his argument further by stating that the concepts of duty and obligation are secondary to – and driven by – that which increases happiness and diminishes harmful outcomes to the rest of society.

So we ask again: how did we manage to reach the point of believing that retrieving every degenerate every time is a bright idea?

The knee-jerk answer might be, of course, that we do what we are expected to do. We respond to and manage the situation of whomever happens to be at the other end of the 911 call.

Some will argue that we do so because civilized society values human life. But that point remains seriously flawed. It is more accurate to accede we have always hung a dubious price tag on any stranger's right to exist. The unrelenting fact is we already value some lives while disregarding others. We already play God. We celebrate the sanctity of the heartbeat, until we are told somebody somewhere ought to be executed. We are strong proponents for child protection, yet overwhelmingly favor fetal death in the realm of abortions. We say it is wrong to kill, unless our leaders tell us people we don't even know, in a far off place we have never seen, ought to be bombed into oblivion by a military action we can neither valuate nor quantify.

Genetic scientists point out there exists an evolutionary struggle on the cellular level between competing sets of co-evolving genes. They believe these genes constantly redesign themselves to defeat each other, in the never-ending leverage to survive. One need not be particularly astute to recognize precisely the same antagonistic dynamic exists within most every U.S. city. We have burgeoning, diverse populations in finite spaces. We spawn rapidly growing volumes of teenagers acting out appalling violence. The ever-growing pockets of fomenting resentment have no choice but to generate a toxic environment. The scientific specialty of *brain plasticity* tells us that changes in the environment create changes in the neural pathways of the brain. As negative behavior socially accumulates, mutations within some brains invariably short circuit rational thinking. The subsequent incivility and inhumanity we see today – even in grade school classrooms – quite naturally pass on to the next generation, guaranteeing a constant withering of human decency; first as sub-cultural tendencies; eventually as a species commonality. By rescuing hellions who would have died 200 years ago, we are ensuring the bad eggs will certainly – by all measurable criteria – live to out breed the well-adjusted.

At some point in America's future, we envision a sea-change in what law-abiding citizenry will tolerate. They just might demand those governing the masses seek peace by inflicting ever more painful consequences. We suspect they will do so in part by once again acknowledging the unflinching laws of nature that have been so respected in the past – one of which is this:

"Specific elimination of maladapted individuals from a population is natural selection."

So, the logical corollary with regards to EMS becomes clear. Our headstrong course to save the "maladapted" along with everyone else, flies in the face of preordained, universal fundamentals. It is equivalent to not eliminating bacteria that, say, poison a water source, out of a twisted reverence for germs' right to life.

In the end, rescue is – is it not? – *the* diamond standard of health care and the acme of human decency. But let us be clear. By sheer definition, EMS manifestly engenders the perfect societal Catch-22. Acts we consider altruistic increase the survival and reproduction of societal evil-doers. Thus, their penchant for misconduct will assuredly spread through the population via natural selection. Evolution – as nearly as can be seen – holds no ethical code nor does it appear to seek ethical consequence. As ample proof, between surfers and sharks, nature reveals a remarkably unequivocal indifference.

Someone brighter than we said that rescue comes from a God-shaped hole in the human fabric, in an attempt to make things right. To our mind, saving a singular life in a singular instance is the epitome of noble behavior – humanity at its finest. Individuals, cases by case, benefit. Yet society, in the aggregate, often suffers. One by one we win. Collectively, we are losing. Why? Simple as soup. We are saving life-forms whom nature throughout the millennia would have otherwise relegated to a befitting and a socially healthier demise. We are – and Satan is in the minutia – degrading the human herd.

Immutable Law # 10

Much of rescue as we know it is inherently insane. It contradicts natural law.

"So what are we trying to overthrow? The target is a health care system that has evolved to serve the interests of those who work in the system. It is a system caught up in the need for profit. It is characterized by many ills, including ineffectiveness, waste, inefficiency, patient waiting, disorganization, disinterest, harm to patients, self-interest and inequity. In effect, it is a stupid system.

What we are doing is a recipe for failure. Only fundamental change will cure its ills. The fact that most of its people are smart, dedicated, caring and good, working within a frustrating system in spite of its flaws, is a national tragedy."

—Donald M. Berwick, MD
Founder, Institute for Healthcare Improvement

FINAL THOUGHTS

Doctor Jeffery MacDonald, found guilty of butchering his family of girls with an ice pick and a bed board, did not turn this Paramedic into a heretic. But he certainly planted the first seed.

Bearing witness to a career full of other physicians who have primped and pilfered, murdered and maimed their way through society – some properly punished, many not – was not the deal breaker, either. But it did plant more seeds.

When a highly respected base-hospital allows a scamp MD on an emergency scene to set a course of non-treatment that guarantees patient death – those seeds become well-fertilized.

When a county EMS system threatens to pull a Paramedic's license because he provides the best possible transportation for head-injured Girl Scouts, such a preposterous mind-bend fuels more than a little skepticism. Thus, the seeds begin to sprout.

A noble profession tolerating the abhorrent propensity to fake patient charts while pretending it does not, stimulates those sprouts of skepticism to seek magnetic North.

When 10 dozen drunken physicians at a medical conference can actually kill a heart patient and then fly back home to their constituency; hire a law firm and sue the Paramedics for 'interference' . . .

When psychiatrists are allowed to churn out byzantine gassiness in the name of healthcare to finance their country club memberships . . .

That hospitals gain enormous wealth by their own mistakes . . .

When pharmaceutical giants are allowed to function as drug providers even after being fined billions upon billions of dollars for lying . . .

When the United States of America ranks somewhere between 29th-37th on the planet in significant health care outcomes . . .

That my colleagues will gladly clamber over alligators to save a life, only to quiver in their boots in the presence of incompetent, unethical doctors . . .

When the *Center for Disease Control* can shroud millions of treatment-related deaths deep within the amphigory of statistical data, and then possess the unmitigated audacity to frighten the public by dangling the flu ghost . . .

That countless thousands of citizens are popping expensive pills because cutie pie drug reps have mastered the dupe-the-doc routine . . .

That the *American Medical Association* vigorously opposes your right to access the *National Practitioner Data Bank*'s bad doctor files, so that . . .

Medical maniacs like Kermit Gosnell and Earl Bradley and Peter LaFuria and Ali Salim and John D. Ott and William H. Ayres and Ivan C. Namihas – barbarians all – can continue for years with their macabre fun and games . . .

Then . . . *then*, the tree of heresy becomes at last full-grown, and being of sound health, recoils from the unrelenting strain of madness afoot. How out of focus must the mind's eye be, to not perceive the dystopian bubble in which Paramedics function? A rescuer can lose a license by saving a life. Yet we tolerate a domain where MDs act out their rogue 'Nestor-5' robotic mischief with such frequency, that theirs is the only profession to possess its very own, newly minted legal term for their degreed caterwauling: *Disruptive Physician*. Other than possibly "going postal" what other occupation holds bragging rights to that achievement? And surrounding these bezonians are techs and nurses, medics and administrators, dutifully falling into line like Stepford Wives, mute to the core. In the strangest of any possible world, the cult of medicine has anointed itself the savior of humanity, even as it will almost certainly kill 2,000,000 citizens by the year 2030. And its engines burn with such visceral fervor that it scares the hell out of this medic, as it certainly ought to scare you.

Simply put, when a veteran rescuer no longer trusts the people he turns patients over to, then it is time to step away. When a Paramedic realizes that his or her partners are too ethically feeble to take a stand in the presence of patient homicide, it is time to acknowledge that one can be too culturally dissimilar to remain. I can no longer in good conscious take the tack of my peers, casually ignoring the horrors many of our patients will be subjected to, as soon as we deliver them to the hurt locker. The system has bullied its membership into believing that anything less than blind and silent support is blasphemy. I, on the other hand, prefer clarity to mind-numbing acquiescence. When you actually believe that drugs are not our salvation at all, but very possibly the downfall of society; when you accept that the credit for human health and longevity goes to advances in better food and clean water and hygiene and sewage disposal over the last 200 years – and not physicians and not vaccines; when you stand convinced that a high grade-point average is the last good reason to select a doctor – then there is likely no place in the EMS system for this medical mugwump.

Even Rod Serling, in the end, could take only so much of the *Twilight Zone*. Or perhaps he fooled us all, and continues to explore its baffling hallways.

But who knows? Maybe more lives are yet to be pried from the jaws of death by this rescuer – granted, in a less scintillating arena – by teaching and lecturing, writing and bloviating. That's a pleasant change of direction after a career chock full of inane politics and never-ending gore, don't you think? So if you don't mind, I'll choose to hang onto that for a while.

Be safe out there. Stay vigilant. And thank you for listening.

❖

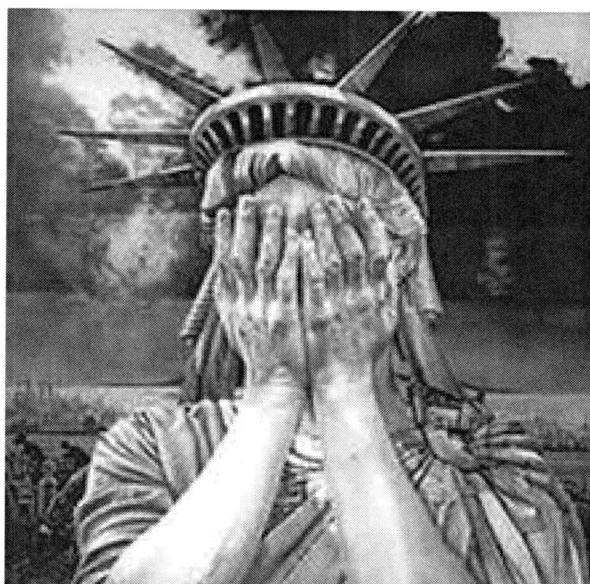

Doesn't true bravery start by simply speaking up?

A Few American Heroes

Not many books are written in a vacuum and this one certainly wasn't. Here are some terrific people who contributed in ways large and small. We suspect true heroes are those who keep close to the ethical compass; find ways to embrace what they do while changing what they can; and remain both vigilant and skeptical. These are the ones who made this book happen even when they didn't know it:

The original *Solana Beach Fire* medics who trained me in phase-three:

Pat Morgan
Dan Ring
Paul Sargent
Jeff Smith
Mike Warner
Dave Weston

And along the way, some fascinating, mind-opening others . . .

Alan Alda, Actor, Director, Author
Gordy Anderson, original San Diego EMT Class 1; Hartson

Ambulance
Paul Anka, Entertainer
Marcia Angell MD, Senior Lecturer, Social Medicine, Harvard
Thea Barsalou, Paramedic, RN, Resuscitative Outcomes Consortium UCSD
Terry Bench, former Medical-legal Editor
Donald Berwick MD, former President, Institute for Healthcare Improvement
Kevin Bacon, Actor
J.B. Brown, EMT, Deputy Sheriff, San Francisco Bay area
Shannon Brownlee, Senior Vice President, the Lown Institute
Corey "Chip" Cheney, Fire Captain, Escondido
Mike Danko, Esq. Aviation Law Monitor
Sean Degnan MD, Cosmetic Dermatology
Thom Dick, Paramedic, Author, Mentor
Joe Dolphin, former President, Medevac Incorporated
Arnold Dorsey, (Engelbert Humperdinck) Entertainer
Chuck Dovey, first San Diego EMS Operations Manager
Randy Easter, EMS Director, McPherson Kansas
David Fish, President, Management Associates, Inc.
Rick Foehr, Paramedic, Director, EMSTA College
Crystal Gayle, Singer, All-around Sweet Person
Charles Glassman MD, Author, Radio Host, Killer Healthcare
Kelly Grayson, Paramedic & Author
Ms. Daryl Hannah, Actress, Activist
William Heisel, Investigative Reporter, Reporting on Health.org
Mary Beth Kellenbarger BSN, former Paramedic Coordinator, Sharp Hospital
Lucian Leape MD, National Patient Safety Foundation
Alan Levine, Researcher; Coordinator, more than 100 patient safety studies
Jacqueline Marcell, Guest Speaker, Author, Radio Host
Robert S. Mendelsohn MD, Physician and Author
Chris Olsen, Paramedic, San Diego County
Gwen Olsen, Pharmaceutical activist, Author
Theresa Oswald, Health Minister, Manitoba Canada

Jerry S. Parr, United States Secret Service (retired)
Barry Silbaugh MD, American College of Physician Executives
Marianne Skolek, Investigative Reporter, Salem-News
Donna Sinclair, President, "Kids on the Block," San Diego
Eric J. Topol, Editor-in-Chief, Medscape
Dennis Quaid, Actor, Patient Safety Advocate
Michael Quitugua, Firefighter/Paramedic, Poway Fire Department
Walt & Virginia Weatherly, California
Pete Wilson, former Governor, State of California
Sidney Wolfe MD, Public Citizen, Co-founder, Health Research Group

❖

In Memoriam

Some of the finest, most supportive people I've known are gone now. Among them are Ken & Juanita McDonald. Here are some others who deserve to be remembered:
Sonny Bono, U.S. Representative, Entrepreneur, Entertainer
Ray Conniff, musical composer, the Ray Conniff Singers
Catherine "Kit' Campion MD, Hoag Hospital Newport Beach
Chris Douglas, Paramedic, Palm Desert California
Tom Fears, NFL Hall of Fame Coach and Palm Desert resident
Cheryl Gibbs, Coroner Investigator, Oakland
Katrina Kish, Flight Nurse, Mercy Air, California
Hilary Koprowski MD, Director, Wistar Institute, Philadelphia
Major W. McBee, Narcotics Advisory Administration, DEA, Southeast Asia
Robert S. Mendelsohn MD
Jerald Miller, Flight Medic, Mercy Air
Margie Nerney, BSN, Paramedic Coordinator, San Diego
Judy Ritchie, BSN, Paramedic Coordinator, Chula Vista

❖

How safe is a career in rescue? You tell us. What follows is a list of my EMS colleagues who have lost their lives, incredibly, just since we sat down to write this book:

EMT Billie J. Grills, 37, on-duty brain hemorrhage, Kentucky
EMS Pilot Ted Caffarel, 59, air ambulance crash, west Texas
Lt. Tim Byrd, 46, collapsed after a drowning-recovery mission, Tennessee
EMT Joseph R. Barlow, 57, head-on ambulance collision, Tennessee
Flight Nurse Sharen Falkener, 46, air ambulance crash, west Texas
Paramedic Gerald Hammer, 62, collapsed after his EMS shift, Indiana
EMT Casey Steenland, 33, carbon monoxide poisoning while on duty, Texas
Paramedic Ruben Berrios, 47, lung complications from the World Trade Center
EMT Mark B. Davis, 25, shot and killed by a patient, New York
EMT Barry Nagle, 66, cardiac arrest while driving an ambulance, Pennsylvania
Flight Nurse James "Jim" Dillow, 35, REACT Team, helicopter crash, Illinois
EMT Melissa Greenhagen, 37, shot and killed in hospital parking lot, Montana
Paramedic Thomas Widcamp, 38, high-wind injuries, Louisiana
Flight Nurse Tracy Chambers, 42, air ambulance crash, West Texas
Fire/Medic Debra Cole, 40, a brain aneurysm on duty, Maine
Doctor Luis Bonilla, 49, Organ Transplant Team, helicopter crash, Florida
EMT Matthew Pellettere, 37, collapsed while on duty, New Jersey
EMT Timothy "Kyle" Southern, 21, ambulance crash, Virginia
EMT Joseph V. Schiumo, 47, lung complications from the World Trade Center
Specialist E. Hoke Smith, 68, Organ Transplant Team, helicopter crash, Florida
Paramedic Raymond B. Allison, 52, ambulance crash, Texas
EMT David J. Gundel, 50, ambulance crash into a tree, Indiana
Justin M. Hueston, 22, vehicle collision, Missouri

Fire Chief Mickey Yates, 47, crash en route to a rescue, Mississippi
Flight Nurse Karen M. Hollis, 48, REACT Team, helicopter crash, Illinois
Paramedic Joshua Weissman, 33, a fall during a rescue, Virginia
EMT William Martin, 56, collapsed during on emergency case, New Jersey
Search & Rescue Tech Ray Shriver, 63, helicopter crash, Wyoming
Paramedic Sarah Nodurft, 27, collapsed during a rescue, West Virginia
EMT Richard Poorman, 52, of West Union
Paramedic Michael Smith, 57, broken neck on duty, Connecticut
EMT Mark Kinder, 26, ambulance crash, West Virginia
EMS Student Cody King, 21, ambulance crash, Ohio
Paramedic Peter Carbonneau, 51, collapsed during a rescue, Maine
EMT Leigh Hebb, 53, ambulance crash, West Virginia
Nurse Andrew "Andy" Olesen, 65, REACT Team, air ambulance crash, Illinois
EMT Belinda Rivers, 43, ambulance crash, South Carolina
Paramedic David Restuccio, 58, ambulance crash, New York
Paramedic Raymond B. Allison, 52, ambulance crash, Texas
EMS Pilot Gene Grell, 56, helicopter crash, Iowa
EMT Timothy C McCormick, 24, ambulance crash, Indiana
Tech. David Hines, 57, Organ Transplant Team, helicopter crash, Florida
EMT Keith Chipepo, 30, ambulance crash, New Jersey
Paramedic Chris Staggs, 35, ambulance crash, West Virginia
EMT Ethan Amsbaugh, 22, ambulance crash, Pennsylvania
Paramedic Joseph Guilmette, 33, Massachusetts
Robert D. Hanes, 51, ambulance crash, Nebraska
Paramedic Brittany M. Despins, 22, hit by car on rescue scene, Michigan
Flight Nurse Shelly Lair-Langenbau, 44, helicopter crash, Iowa
EMT Teresa Ann Davis, 44, ambulance crash, Georgia

Paramedic Russell Piehl, 48, helicopter crash, Iowa
EMT Eric Monty, 45, ambulance crash, New York
Fire/Medic James Brooks, 62, collapsed on duty, Maryland
Paramedic Randall H. Whiddon, 56, ambulance crash, Georgia
EMT Esteban Bahema, 24, struck by a vehicle on the freeway, San Diego
Paramedic Cody Medley, 22, ambulance crash, Indianapolis
EMT Wesley Hostetter, 30, ambulance crash, Pennsylvania
Paramedic Brian Schimpf, 33, EMS vehicle roll-over injuries, Colorado
Flight Paramedic Herman Dobbs, 40, helicopter crash, Kentucky
Flight Nurse Jesse Jones, 28, helicopter crash, Kentucky
Pilot Eddy Sizemore, 62, helicopter crash, Kentucky
EMT Terry Lynne Niles, 50, collapsed on an emergency, New Hampshire
Flight Nurse Christopher Denning, 41, helicopter crash, Oklahoma
EMT Wilbur Fraenzel, 30, collapsed on duty, Virginia
Pilot Mark A. Montgomery, 47, helicopter crash, Oklahoma
Paramedic Chris Douglas, 41, struck by a vehicle, California
EMT Thomas Gruen, 46, ambulance crash, Pennsylvania
Fire/EMT Wayne Jeffers, 64, collapsed on duty, Alabama
Fire/Medic Chad Null, 33, collapsed after an EMS call, Indiana
Paramedic Paul Boyer, 54, ambulance crash into a tree, North Carolina
Paramedic Supervisor Dale R. Long, 48, ambulance collision, Vermont
Flight Paramedic Shawn Baker, 42, collapsed on duty, Ohio
EMT Sherry Pettit, 40, struck and killed by a city bus on duty, Ohio
EMT Steve Lovato, 30, shot and killed by a burn patient, New Mexico

❖

Medics see an awful lot of death – including each other's – and I've seen more than most. When the following citizens left this earth, I was there:

Billy Adams, San Pedro
Judy Allen, Los Angeles
Don Ashcroft, Sacramento
Bryce Banner, Los Angeles
Daniel Lawrence Balson, Encino
Leonard Barr, Loomis
Mary Beard, Sacramento
Frank Becwar, Fair Oaks
Robert Benner, Thousand Oaks
Sue Benner, Thousand Oaks
David Bernard, Santa Monica
Paula Blake, Playa del Rey
Barbara Boisselle, Los Angeles
Karen Borzewski, San Diego
Charles Bren, Los Angeles
Ronald Henry Burkley, Manhattan Beach
Arnold Lee Califf, Poway
Joseph Reed Canavin, Andover, Mass.
Hood Cheney, Dallas
Lynn Cherry, San Diego
Pauleen Colarich, Concord
Martha J. Coleman, San Diego
Alberico Coluzzi, Los Angeles
Richard W. Conway, San Diego
Carol Cook, Rolling Hills
Christine Davie, Carlsbad
Lisa Denise Davis, Lakeside
Olga R. de Huante, San Diego
Timothy DeLuca, Aptos
Gerri Dixon, Los Angeles
Janet Dolson, Inglewood
James W. Dormer, San Diego
Jay Drotman, Santa Monica
John Dumas, Los Angeles
Kirk C. Dutton, Los Angeles
Amancio Elizaga, San Diego

Javier Escalante, Sacramento
Jonathon Falk, Los Angeles
Michael Fitzgerald, San Diego
Perry Flashman, Culver City
Kate Fons, San Diego
Gail Michele Forsyth, San Diego
Gary Fox, Culver City
Robert E. Fox, Pilot, La Mesa
William Francis, Sacramento
James Gallagher, Bakersfield
Maureen Gallagher, Bakersfield
Jay Gilroy, San Francisco
Robert Guerrero, Sacramento
Jacob Joseph Gustinic, Marina Del Rey
Lewis Hayden, San Diego
Steve Henry, Sacramento
Richard Hight, Citrus Heights
Ric Horne, Glendale
Jack Irwin, Sacramento
Barbara Jackson, Los Angeles
Nellie Jackson, Sacramento
Andria Jacobson, Belmont Shores
Neil Howard Jagoba, Framingham, Mass.
George Johnson, Thousand Oaks
Lee H. Johnson, La Jolla
David L. Jolliffee, Los Angeles
Valerie Kantor, Pacific Palisades
Jimmie A. Kelly, Savannah, Ga.
Colleen A. Kepler, San Diego
Farrell Kimball, Sacramento
Allan Lebow, Los Angeles
Wayne Allen Levin, Beverly Hills
Robert Levine, San Diego
David Loeb, Santa Monica
Rosalia Lococa, Santee;
Earl Lohnes, Niantic, Conn.

Brian T. MacLean, San Diego
Jesus Macias, Hawthorne
Gil A. Marcoux, San Diego
Andrew Martin, Malibu
Louise T. Martin, San Diego
Thomas Masker, Monterey
Debbi McCarthy, Vista
James F. McFeron, Pilot, Escondido
Joseph McMasters, Sacramento
Joann Metzler, Thunder Bay, Ontario, Canada
Charles Miller, Davis
Samuel Molinaro, El Cajon
Gary Moore, Sacramento
Whilhelmina Mottola, San Diego
Kenji Nakanishi, Santa Monica
Spencer B. Nelson, Pilot, off-duty, Escondido
Betty Nunn, Hayward
Robert Oshiro, Sacramento
Lynn Owens, Coronado
Gary Patterson, Highland
Bernard Perez, Shingle Springs
Jeffrey J. Pesses, Los Angeles
Burt Pierce, Rancho Palos Verdes
Richard Plaskoff, Los Angeles
Anthony Poli, San Diego
Gary Ponnells, Citrus Heights
Muhamed Quaffae, Alshwah, Kuwait
Bob Ramirez, Lennox
Leo Reeder, Pacific Palisades
Ronnie Resnick, Los Angeles
Francis Resnick, Los Angeles
Joseph Rigney, Downey
Randy Ryckman, Santa Monica
Don C. St. Germain, San Diego
George Saunders, Rancho Palos Verdes
Maria C. Scavia, La Mesa

Dave Schmidt, Sacramento
Ralph Schuerler, Sacramento
Bennett Schwartz, Culver City
James Seaman, Manhattan Beach
Nerene Fay Seaton, Bakersfield
Gail Lynn Shapiro, San Diego
Robert Sinclair Silver, Marina Del Rey
Kirt Smith, Palo Alto
Walter Smith, Citrus Heights
Roger Smith, Waukesha, Wis.
Herb L. Stewart, Monterey
Jim Stinnett, Los Angeles
Michael Sulit, Del Mar
James Taggart, Palos Verdes
Azmi David Taha, Vista
Allen Tetelman, Los Angeles
Maxine Thweatt, Manhattan Beach
Daniel Bruce Urdahl, San Diego
Martin J. Wahne, Flight Engineer, San Diego
Roger W. Walsh, Solana Beach
William White, Lakeside
Kevin Wholey, Santa Monica
Jane Whyte-Spitz, Bonita
Jeff Wilson, Los Angeles
Lawrence Wilson, Sacramento
Tom Womack, El Cajon
Dee Anne Young, El Cajon
David Lee Boswell, Camp Pendleton
Martin Kazy Jr., San Diego
Amy Bolick, San Diego
Nancy Stout, San Diego
Robert Stout, San Diego
Lela Todd, San Diego
Derek Walker, San Diego
Sherry Walker, San Diego
Darlene Watkins, San Diego

McDonald's Massacre Victims

I put a hand on each face and wept for these, too:

Elsa Herlinda Borboa-Firro,19, McDonald's employee
Neva Denise Caine, 22, McDonald's manager)
Michelle Deanne Carncross,18
María Elena Colmenero-Silva,19
David Flores Delgado, 11
Gloria López González, 23
Omar Alonso Hernández, 11
Blythe Regan Herrera, 31
Matao Herrera, 11
Paulina Aquino López, 21, employee
Margarita Padilla, 18, employee
Claudia Pérez, 9
Jose Rubén Lozano Pérez, 19
Carlos Reyes, 8 months
Jackie Lynn Wright Reyes, 18
Victor Maxmillian Rivera, 25
Arisdelsi Vuelvas Vargas, 31
Hugo Luis Velazquez Vasquez, 45
Laurence Herman "Gus" Versluis, 62
Aida Velazquez Victoria, 69
Miguel Victoria-Ulloa, 74

Palm Springs Bus Tragedy

Richard A. Gonzales, 23, Colton Ca. bus driver
Laurel McDaniel, 30, Norcross Ga., chaperone
Zoe Jackson, 15, Sangerville Me.,
Tammy Murray, 15, Detroit
Jennifer Barnum, 16, Rochester Hills, Mich.
Vicki Powell, age unknown, Fairburn, Ga., advisor
Doneta Schaeffer, age unknown, Davenport, Iowa, advisor

And Mr. Anthony Ward, 54, who collapsed at a Palm Springs medical convention and was killed by several dozen drunk physicians.

Support Material and Extra Reading

Author note: Each legal case mentioned within this text is verified by a minimum of three sources. We include no case, nor do we mention any name, which has not been repeatedly documented. Criminal cases found herein are detailed only after guilt was determined. All cases are verifiable through state and federal court records. They can be found in law enforcement advisories, such as *FBI*; state district attorney websites; the *DEA* and local police department press releases.

❖

Chapter One:

Return to Dwight and Nile: the Crash of PSA Flight 182
Video documentary, Director David Fresina, Natascot Films

The McDonald's Massacre
YouTube News footage, multiple providers

One Killed in 100-Car Pile-up in California
Google News clip

Chapter Two:

Rescuers Stood by While Man Drowned in Alameda
SF Gate website news

Elderly Woman Dies after Nurse Refuses to Give Her CPR
ABC News go.com

Girl Scout Bus Accident Kills 7 near Palm Springs
Deseret News.com

Chapter Three:

Bad Blood: Doctor-Nurse Behavior Problems Impact Patient Care
Carrie Johnson, American College of Healthcare Executives, ACHE.org

Chapter Four:

Controversies in Prehospital Care
David M. Lemonick, MD

Golden Hour and Other Myths
Mike Danko, Aviation Law Monitor

Misuse of Lights and Sirens
Siren Facts.com

Study: Medical Sirens Overused
Tim Bonfield, Cincinnati Enquirer

Use of Lights and Sirens
Med-X Medical Services.com

Chapter Five:

CPR is Less Effective than We Think
George Lundberg, MD

'Do Not Resuscitate' Orders
Cleveland Clinic.org

Does CPR Save Lives?
Doctor Skeptic website

How Do Doctors and Non-physicians Want to Die?
Lisa Wade, PhD research, Society Pages.org

How Doctors Choose to Die
Ken Murray, MD essay in The Guardian

Sudden Death and the Myth of CPR
Stefan Timmermans

Chapter Six:

Accountability
Dr. Marty Makary

A Sea of Broken Hearts: Patient Rights in a Dangerous, Profit-Driven Health Care System"
Dr. John T. James, PhD

Chasing Zero: Winning the War on Health care Harm
TMIT Research documentary

The Checklist Manifesto
Atul Gawande, MD

Confessions of a Surgeon: The Good, the Bad, and the Complicated
Paul A. Ruggieri

Death by Modern Medicine: Seeking Safer Solutions
Carolyn Dean

Doctors Perform Thousands of Unnecessary Surgeries
Health Impact News website

First, Do No Harm: The Cure for Medical Malpractice
Ira E. Williams, DDS

A Gynecologist's Second Opinion
William Parker, MD, medical investigator

Hospitals and Health
Abram Hoffer, Andrew Saul
Andrew Saul co-authors a book on the issue of safeguarding your health while in the hospital

Hospital Medical Errors Now the Third Leading Cause of Death in the U.S.
Llene MacDonald, FierceHealthCare.com

Infections with 'Nightmare Bacteria' on the Rise in U.S. Hospitals
Rob Stein, public health contributor, NPR.org

Internal Bleeding: The Truth Behind America's Terrifying Epidemic of Medical Mistakes
Robert M. Wachter, MD

Medically Caused Death in America
Jon Rappoport Interview with Doctor Barbara Starfield
NoMoreFakeNews.com

Medical Errors and Medical Narcissism
John Banja, PhD

Nip/Tuck Nightmare: The Dangerous New World or Cosmetic Surgery
Roxanne Patel Shepelavy, Fox News website health contributor

Survive Your Hospital Stay
Consumer Reports

Thousands of Doctors Practicing Despite Errors, Misconduct
Peter Eisler, Barbara Hansen, USA Today Healthcare Investigation

When Healthcare Makes You Sick
A 'USA Today' Investigative series

Why the 'Best' Hospitals Might also be the Most Dangerous
Shannon Brownlee, Time Magazine online

World Health Organization's Ranking of the World's Health Systems
The Patient Factor website

Chapter Seven:

The Dark Side of Medicine: Writing Lies into the Medical Record
Maurice Bernstein, MD, Bioethics discussion

Dishonesty in Medicine Revisited
Herbert L. Fred, MD, NCBI.gov website

Doctors Approved Fake Patient Charts in $200M Medicare Fraud
Sandra Yin, Reporter, FierceHealthCare.com

The Treatment Trap
Rosemary Gibson, Janardan P Singh

Firms Raided in Massive Workers' Comp Probe
Articles.LAtimes.com/1993-07-01

Chapter Eight:

Before You Take that Pill
J. Douglas Bremner, MD

Broken Brains or Wounded Hearts
Ty Colbert, MD

Diary of a Legal Drug Dealer
K. L. Carlson

Drugs for Life: How Pharmaceutical Companies Define Our Health
Joseph Dumit

Hard Sell: The Evolution of a Viagra Salesman."
Jamie Reidy

Overdosed America
John Anderson reveals the extent of perverted clinical drug trials

Overtreated: Why Too Much Medicine Is Making Us Sicker and Poorer
Shannon Brownlee

Pharmageddon
David Healy, MD

Chapter Nine:

Bad Medicine: Doctors Doing Harm since Hippocrates
David Wootten, Professor of History, University of New York

Blind Eye: The Terrifying Story of a Doctor Who Got Away With Murder
James B. Stewart

Brief History of Bad Medicine
Robert Youngson

Cracked: Why Psychiatry is Doing More Harm than Good
James Davies, PhD

"Doc": The Rape of the Town of Lovell
Jack Olsen

Doctor Dealer: The Rise & Fall of an All American Boy
Mark Boden

Fatal Vision
Joe McGinniss

The Good Doctor
Wensley Clarkson

Gosnell's Babies
Steve Volk

Murder in Wellesley
Tom Farmer, Marty Foley

On the Take
Jerome P. Kassirer, MD

Chapter Ten:

Kant in the Classroom
Manchester University website

Hobbes Moral and Political Philosophy
Stanford Encyclopedia of Philosophy

Utilitarianism.com
John Stuart Mill
George Sher

Utilitarian Ethics Essays
The Wise Geek website

❖

A few other excellent resources

Anatomy of an Epidemic: Magic Bullets, Psychiatric Drugs, and the Astonishing Rise of Mental Illness in America
Robert Whitaker

Before You Take that Pill
J. Douglas Bremner, MD

Collateral Damage: A Patient, a New Procedure, and the Learning Curve
Dan Walter

Condition Critical
Echo Heron, BSN

Death by Medicine
Gary Null, PhD

Doctor Yourself: Natural Healing That Works
Andrew W. Saul, Carol Rosenberg

Elder Rage
Ms. Jacqueline Marcell

The Emperor's New Drugs: Exploding the Antidepressant Myth
Irving Kirsch

Escape Fire: Designs for the Future of Health Care
Donald Berwick, MD

Flu Vaccine: Something to Sneeze At
Roman Bystrianyk

Health Care Regulation in America
Robert I. Field

Heart Frauds
Charles T. McGee exposes some serious mythology

Hippocrates (Medicine and Culture)
Jacques Jouanna, Malcolm DeBevoise

How we do Harm
Otis Brawley, MD, Chief Medical Officer, American Cancer Society; Paul Goldberg

Influence: The Psychology of Persuasion
Robert Cialdini. PhD

Medicine in Denial
Lawrence Reed

Politics in Healing
Daniel Haley

Saving Normal: An Insider's Revolt Against Out-Of-Control Psychiatric Diagnosis, DSM5, Big Pharma, and the Medicalization of Ordinary Life
Allen Frances, MD

Seeking Sickness: Medical Screening and the Misguided Hunt for Disease
Alan Cassels

Should I Be Tested for Cancer?
H. Gilbert Welch, Evidence of harm in excessive testing

Shyness: How Normal Behavior Became a Sickness
Christopher Lane

Side Effects: a Prosecutor, a Whistleblower, and a Bestselling Anti-depressant on Trial
Alison Bass

Toxic Psychiatry; Talking Back to Prozac
Peter Breggin

The Truth about Drug Companies
Marcia Angell, MD, Former Editor-in-Chief, *New England Journal of Medicine*

The $800 Million Pill
Merrill Goozner

To Err Is Human: Building a Safer Health System
Linda Kohn, Janet Corrigan, Molla Donaldson, Editors

Unhinged: The Trouble with Psychiatry—A Doctor's Revelations about a Profession in Crisis
Daniel Carlat

Waking Up Blind
Tom Harbin, MD

Whole New Life: an Illness and a Healing
Reynolds Price

❖

It was never our intent to insult the 'feel good' works of EMS. Some of them are pretty darn good:

Bringing Out the Dead
Downloadable movie

EMS: The Job of Your Life
Devin Kerins

EMT: Beyond the Lights & Sirens
Pat Ivey

En Route: A Paramedic's Stories
Steven "Kelly" Grayson

Into the Breach: a Year of Life and Death in EMS
J.A. Karam

A Paramedic's Diary
Stuart Gray

A Paramedic's Story: Life and Death and Everything in Between
Steven "Kelly" Grayson

Paramedic: On the Front Lines
Peter Canning

Rescuing Providence
Michael Morse

Strength, Love & Ambulances
Rebecca Stone, EMT

Weep Not, My Wanton
Maggie Dubris

❖

A few terrific websites

Accident Archives
U.S. Department of Labor

AllNurses.com

Ambulance Driver Files.com

Archives of Internal Medicine
Bioethics Discussion on blogspot.com

Choosing Wisely

Citizens for Patient Safety

ConsumerHealthChoices.org/

Dartmouth Atlas

Doctor Discipline Database

Doctor Yourself.com

DrivetoSurvive.org/

Ethicalnag.org

FSMB.org
Federation of State Medical Boards

Harvard.edu/Clinician-Resources

HealthGrades.com

Health-Matrix.net

HospitalSafetyScore.org

Leapfrog Group

ISMP.org
Institute for Safe Medical Practices

KevinMD.com

Medicare.gov/Hospitals-Compared

MedicalMiscreants.com

MedicalAuthorChat.com

Medic Scribe.com

National Practitioner Data Bank

Patient's Checklist

ProPublica Patient Harm

Public Citizen and Health Research Group

Reporting on Health.org

SafePatientProject.org

SafetyLeaders.org

SkepticalScalpel Blog

Street Watch blog

Supporting Safer Health Care.com

RateMDs.com

Rogue Medic website

Vitals.com

WorstPills.org

And of course, the *Paramedic Heretic* website

End

Also by this author:

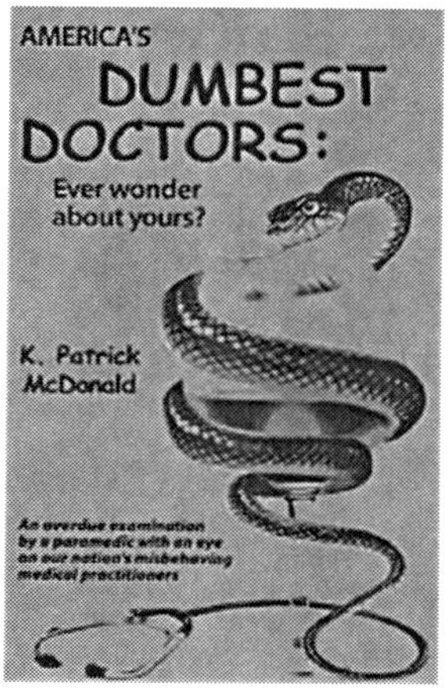

Health care reform? Why not start by simply tossing out the trash?

In this non-fiction study of physician misconduct, we learn for the first time what happens when a rescuer focuses his penlight on the idiocy around him and unleashes 30 years of note-taking.

In *America's Dumbest Doctors*, author McDonald has produced a book that literally no other Paramedic has dared to publish, detailing exactly who the 'bad guys' are: licensed professionals inappropriately held in such high esteem by the public. McDonald, a traditionally trained EMS program graduate of *UCSD School of Medicine* in La Jolla, not only reveals first-hand instances of doctors behaving badly, but includes revelations from nurses, the media, and physicians, who themselves are so often embarrassed by their peers.

Consider the Arizona MD who – while facing 67 counts of sexually abusing his patients – announced in court, "Okay, so I'm not exactly Dr. Marcus Welby." Or take the East Coast doctor who stole a cadaver's hand in order to impress a topless dancer. Or the Tennessee MD who wrote to Bank of America, "This person is dead. She is green and has maggots crawling on her. Stop asking about her status."

A retired chief of medicine from San Diego said this: "McDonald breaks rank and names names. I wish I could report that these are merely a few far-out nutcases. I honestly cannot say that. And this fact alone makes his work, regrettably, important."

The comedy of *America's Dumbest Doctors* will entertain you. The sheer volume of idiocy will educate you. And the moral of the story will probably save lives.

(For more about the book and the subject visit **www.MedicalMiscreants.com**)

CPSIA information can be obtained
at www.ICGtesting.com
Printed in the USA
FSOW01n1113150417
33044FS

9 781457 531804